Bayesian Inference for Partially Identified Models

Exploring the Limits of Limited Data

MONOGRAPHS ON STATISTICS AND APPLIED PROBABILITY

General Editors

F. Bunea, V. Isham, N. Keiding, T. Louis, R. L. Smith, and H. Tong

Monographs on Statistics and Applied Probability 141

Bayesian Inference for Partially Identified Models

Exploring the Limits of Limited Data

Paul Gustafson

University of British Columbia

Vancouver, Canada

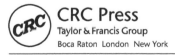

CRC Press
Taylor & Francis Group
Boca Raton   London   New York

CRC Press is an imprint of the
Taylor & Francis Group, an **informa** business

A CHAPMAN & HALL BOOK

CRC Press
Taylor & Francis Group
6000 Broken Sound Parkway NW, Suite 300
Boca Raton, FL 33487-2742

Version Date: 20150211

International Standard Book Number-13: 978-1-4398-6939-0 (Hardback)

Visit the Taylor & Francis Web site at
http://www.taylorandfrancis.com

and the CRC Press Web site at
http://www.crcpress.com

To Reka, Joseph, Lucas, and Anna

Contents

List of Figures

List of Tables

Preface

Back in 2001, two co-authors and I published a paper titled, "Case-Control Analysis with Partial Knowledge of Exposure Misclassification Probabilities." This was motivated as methodology for a practical biostatistical task: to analyze case-control data when the exposure variable is poorly measured, and one has only a rough idea of how poorly. And the task seemed to cry out for Bayesian analysis, since having a rough idea about something is akin to having a prior distribution. However, when embarking on this research, I did not anticipate how interesting it would be (at least to me!) to characterize the behavior of the posterior distribution as the sample size grows. We all learn early on that in well-posed problems the width of the posterior distribution scales with the reciprocal of the square root of the sample size. And we tend to intuit that if we cannot stuff the problem at hand into this "well-posed" (i.e., identified) framework, then we are stuck and should give up. Yet, here was quite a simple and practical problem that did not fit the "root-n" paradigm, but at the same time did not seem to be a hopeless problem. This fascinated me, and I was hooked.

Of course upon digging deeper I realized that I was far from the first to think about these things. In the literature there is a historical, albeit small, trail of foundational papers characterizing identification from a Bayesian perspective. In addition, in the Markov chain Monte Carlo "gold rush" of the 1990s, there were isolated instances of people tackling applied problems in the spirit of: we know this model is not identified, but given the data we can turn the Bayesian computational crank nonetheless, and see what comes out.

Neither of these streams in the literature seemed to emphasize questions of information flow— to what extent does the posterior distribution narrow as the data accumulate? Under what circumstances will the posterior distribution on the target parameter be usefully narrow versus uselessly wide? This struck me as pretty important, and over the last fourteen years much of my research has been pitched in this direction. What follows in these pages is my attempt to summarize the fruits of these labors.

Directly or indirectly, many people have helped me in pursuing this research agenda and writing this monograph. To avoid arbitrarily dichotomizing a continuous spectrum, I will not thank people by name. Rather, I issue a general "shout out" of thanks to numerous colleagues, collaborators, graduate students (past and present), CRC Press staff members, and, yes, even to all those tough peer reviewers out there. It has been a pleasure to interact with all of you folks in this research domain.

And finally, as ever, I thank my family for their love and support. Since I'm not naming names, I will use instead examples of endearing traits that contribute so much to my life. Thanks to a daughter so organized that sometimes tomorrow's clothes are laid out in "person shape" on her bedroom floor. (How do you put up with the rest of us?) Thanks to a son so eclectic as to have, for instance, an encyclopedic knowledge of football (i.e., soccer) squads and results the world over. (How can you so effortlessly recall scores of matches played before you were born?) Thanks to another son so adventurous as to be "busted" by social media photos of his extreme parkouring exploits. (How did you get to the top of that massive bird statue at Olympic Village, and how could you not think it dangerous?) And so much thanks to a wife so accomplished and caring and generally impressive on the one hand, yet so easily and delightfully distracted by "something shiny over there" on the other. This wonderful crew keeps me on my toes, in a manner with which partially identified models cannot compete!

Guide to Notation

d, d_n	observed data (without/with emphasis on sample size n)
$d^\star, d_n^\star$	observable data (pre-observation, as random variables)
$\theta, \gamma, \lambda, \ldots$	parameters in generic terms
$\theta^\star, \gamma^\star, \lambda^\star, \ldots$	parameters as random variables
$\theta^\dagger, \gamma^\dagger, \lambda^\dagger, \ldots$	true values of parameters
θ	whole parameter vector
$(\phi, \lambda) = h(\theta)$	transparent reparameterization
$\psi = \tilde{g}(\theta) = g(\phi, \lambda)$	scalar parameter of interest
a_{i+}	$\sum_{j=1}^{J} a_{ij}$
$a_{i\bullet}$	$(a_{i1}, \ldots a_{iJ})$
$\pi()$	actual prior and posterior densities
$\pi^*()$	convenience prior and posterior densities
LPD	limiting posterior distribution
PIM	partially identified model
IPPM	identified but possibly misspecified model
■	end of example
★	end of aside

Chapter 1

Introduction

1.1 Identification

What is Identification?

A statistical model postulates how the probability distribution of observable variables depends on unknown parameters. This leads to the possibility of estimating these parameters, after having observed the variables for a sample of units from the population under study. A nice property for a statistical model to possess is that of *identification*. While more technical statements are possible, the intuitive content of identification is that different settings of the parameters cannot produce the same joint probability distribution of the observables. More formally, consider the mapping from the *parameter space*, the set of possible values for the parameters, to the set of possible distributions for the observables. Identification corresponds to invertibility of this mapping. That is, multiple points in the parameter space never map to the same distribution of observables. When identification holds, nice things happen. Principally, as we collect more data, we can better estimate the distribution of observables. Therefore, under the additional assumption that the mapping is smooth, as well as invertible, this learning translates very directly to learning about the parameters.

Without identification, the situation is much less satisfactory. We can still learn the distribution of observables from the data, but transmuting this information back to the parameter space will be less useful than in the identified case. Consider the extreme case where the distribution of observables is known exactly. This can be regarded as the limiting case as the amount of data, i.e., the size of the sample, goes to infinity. Without identification, this distribution will generally map back to a set of values in the parameter space rather than a single value. Clearly, this is disquieting. Data are generally expensive to collect, but we embark upon scientific studies nonetheless, based on the premise that we can march toward knowledge of "the truth" as we allocate more and more resources toward data acquisition. Without identification, however, we face the cost of obtaining data without the guarantee of a march to certainty. Put more bluntly, with identification lacking, even the collection of data *ad infinitum* will not reveal the actual values of the parameters.

1

Given the appeal of identification and the woe associated with its absence, it is legitimate to ask: why ever bother with statistical models that lack identification? Why not just stick to the nice identified models? To some extent, the statistical community does just that. The overwhelming majority of statistical models proposed in the methodological literature and used in the wider scientific literature are indeed identified models. To understand why it might not be best practice to immediately eliminate nonidentified models from consideration, we need to "drill down" a bit, to discuss both objectives and data availability in some scientific areas where statistical modelling is commonplace.

Observational Studies

In many areas of scientific enquiry, an *observational study* is the common, or perhaps only, study design employed. As the name implies, such a study involves no intervention on units in the study sample. One only observes the values of a suite of variables on these units. To fix ideas, consider a common situation in various health and social science settings. The suite of variables is (Y, X, C), where Y is an "outcome" or "response" variable, X is an "exposure" or "treatment" variable, and C is a collection of "covariates" or "potential confounders." In lay terms, the scientific goal is to assess the extent, if any, to which X influences Y. As an example of a situation where this scientific goal is well founded, say X encodes an individual's level of exposure to a possibly harmful substance, and Y indicates whether or not the person contracts a particular disease. In terms of statistical modelling, some form of regression model can be employed, capturing the conditional distribution of Y given X and C. Such a model will generally be identified: there are no serious impediments to data in the form of observations from the joint distribution of (Y, X, C) revealing parameters describing the conditional distribution of $(Y|X, C)$.

Threats to Validity

Unfortunately, there are a number of "threats to validity" for observational studies. One is the threat of *unobserved confounding*. Roughly put, the conditional distribution of $(Y|X, C)$ only reveals the *causal* influence of X on Y provided that C contains *all* confounding variables, i.e., all variables that might influence both X and Y. If this is the case, then theory supports a regression model applied to the observational data estimating the same "effect of X on Y" that would be targeted in a study involving intervention, i.e., a randomized trial in which subjects are randomly allocated to different levels of the exposure X. In concept this is wonderful, as we can estimate the effect of *intervening* on X in settings where a study that actually intervenes on X would be impractical or unethical. That is, we can target the "causal" effect of X on Y. In practice it is less wonderful, since there is no algorithm or empirical check for whether the potential confounders selected for measurement in the study do indeed include all the actual confounding variables. Put another way, say that C indeed contains all actual confounders; however, we may only be able to identify and measure a subset of them. Say $C = (C_1, C_2)$, where we can observe C_1 but not C_2. On the modelling side we are obliged to consider a parameterized model describing (Y, X, C_1, C_2), in order to go after the causal effect of X on Y. This then induces a model for the distribution of the observables (Y, X, C_1) given the parameters. Generally, unless very much is known or assumed about the relationship of C_2 with the observable variables, this model will lack identification.

A different threat to validity is that of poor measurement. For instance, say that best efforts to assess the exposure variable, X, produce a variable, X^*, which differs from X for some study subjects. On the modeling side we are still obliged to focus on (Y, X, C) in order to be going after the quantities of real scientific interest, involving the relationship of the actual exposure with the outcome. Moreover, we must additionally model the relationship between the measured exposure X^* and the actual exposure X. The modelling implies a distribution for the observables (Y, X^*, C), but the resulting model may lack identification. There are exceptions, but a general rule would be that the presence of unknown parameters in the relationship between X^* and X renders the model for the observables nonidentified. Barring some further source of information, knowledge of the (Y, X^*, C) distribution is not sufficiently rich to reveal all the salient details of the (Y, X, C) distribution.

Yet another threat to validity is that of selection bias. In the discussion to this point, there has been an implicit assumption that the study sample is representative of the population of interest. Often this comes specifically in the form of assuming the study sample is chosen at random from the population. In many realistic settings, however, it is hard or impossible to ensure that all population members have the same chance of selection. So, whereas random selection would give rise to the joint distribution of (Y, X, C) that is of scientific interest, the actual sampling scheme may induce a different joint distribution of outcome, exposure, and potential confounders. For concreteness, say that $(\tilde{Y}, \tilde{X}, \tilde{C})$ follow this distribution. A now familiar refrain ensues. Unless a lot is known about the mechanics of how the sampling scheme favors some population members over others, learning the joint distribution of $(\tilde{Y}, \tilde{X}, \tilde{C})$ from the observed data will not serve to completely reveal the distribution of (Y, X, C).

The thread between these threats to validity is that they all involve some form of coarsening or corruption of the ideal data we wish we had. We wish we had observations from a random sample of (Y, X, C). What we actually have is observations from a random sample on some corrupted form of the variables, be that (Y, X, C_1), (Y, X^*, C), or $(\tilde{Y}, \tilde{X}, \tilde{C})$. Thus we have a conundrum. The quantities of real scientific interest lie in the joint distribution of the ideal data.

However, a statistical model for the ideal data, combined with a model linking the corrupted data and the ideal data, will typically induce a nonidentified model for the corrupted data. This commonly arises, even if in isolation the model for the ideal data is identified, in the hypothetical context of the ideal data being observable.

On the other hand, while it would typically be straightforward to construct an identified model for the corrupted data directly—say regressing Y on (X, C_1), or Y on (X^*, C), or $\tilde{Y}$ on $(\tilde{X}, \tilde{C})$—the quantities of real scientific interest will not be encoded in such a model. Thus we are forced down the path of investigating what corrupted data can actually tell us about the quantities of scientific interest, despite this corresponding to inference via a nonidentified model. In the hope that at least sometimes corrupted data can tell us something useful, we now make a subtle change in terminology. While this book does indeed focus on statistical models that lack identification, we will tend, in fact, to refer to such models as *partially identified*. In part, this is simply for the sake of a more optimistic label, to avoid the nihilistic-sounding "nonidentified" as a descriptor. But it transpires that there are mathematical quantifications of the extent to which the models we work with literally are identified "in part." Thus we embark upon a voyage around the world of the partially identified model, abbreviated PIM hereafter.

1.2   What is against Us?

Lack of Consistent Estimators

There is no shirking the formidable challenges in drawing inferences based on statistical models that lack identification. We cannot fall back on the nice "textbook" properties of inference based on identified models. To start, we cannot expect *consistent* estimation of target quantities of interest. In many contexts, the property of consistency, whereby a point estimator converges to the correct value of its target as the sample size increases to infinity, is viewed as a minimum hurdle to clear. Estimators not attaining this property are dismissed summarily. When we lack identification, however, we cannot hope for consistency. Typically, multiple values of the target are consistent with the distribution of the observables, so no amount of data can distinguish the actual value of the target from amongst a set of plausible values. It follows immediately that we must view problems lacking identification through a very different lens than we use for their identified counterparts.

Lack of Valid Confidence Intervals

Moving on to interval estimation, in the identified model landscape we seek, and can find, procedures that have the desired frequentist coverage. Say, for instance, that the customary confidence level of 95% is sought. Then we can hope to find a procedure, taking a dataset as input and providing an interval of target values as the output, with the right coverage. That is, if datasets were repeatedly generated under the same parameter values, 95% of these would yield an interval containing the correct value of the target. Moreover, this property applies regardless of which parameter values are considered.

While it can be hard to construct an interval estimator for which this property holds *exactly*, via large-sample theory it is typically easy to engineer procedures with approximately correct frequentist coverage, in an "asymptotic" sense. More formally, with an identified model one can usually construct a procedure for which the probability of covering the target converges to the desired coverage rate as the sample size goes to infinity. As well, whether the coverage is exact or only asymptotic, confidence intervals in most identified model contexts have a predictable regularity: their width scales as the reciprocal of the square-root of sample size. This "root-n" behavior is infused in the statistical ether, particularly via the rule-of-thumb that doubling precision (i.e., halving interval width) requires quadrupling sample size. Succinctly stated, with the luxury of an identified model which happens to be true, typically one enjoys a "root-n march" to the certainty of the correct value of the target.

As we shall see later in this book, when identification is lost, correct frequentist coverage, or even approximately correct coverage asymptotically, is another casualty. We know we cannot expect a root-n march to the right answer, since more than one value of the target is compatible with the distribution of the observables. But, setting aside the issue of how the width of the interval scales with the amount of data, it proves impossible to construct procedures with the right coverage, even in the limiting asymptotic sense. At best we might seek conservative procedures, having a coverage probability that varies with the underlying parameter values but never dips below the desired level.

1.3   What is For Us?

The Bayesian Crank

With the textbook properties of consistent estimation for point estimators and correct frequentist coverage for interval estimators lost, we need to take stock of what, if anything, works *for* us when thinking about inference based on a partially identified model. In terms of a mechanical route to determining parameter estimators, we are still free to adopt a Bayesian point of view. We start with specifying a *prior distribution* for the parameters, representing our knowledge about these parameters in advance of collecting data. Then, once the data are in hand, we can "turn the Bayesian crank" to update prior beliefs into posterior beliefs. That is, Bayes theorem is applied, with the prior distribution as one input, and the likelihood function arising from the statistical model and the data as the other input. The output is the posterior distribution over possible parameter values, representing the post-data knowledge about the parameters. Provided we supply a legitimate probability distribution as the prior distribution, Bayes theorem will output a legitimate probability distribution as the posterior distribution. This is the case *whether or not the model is identified*. Thus the Bayesian approach to inference is at least applicable in the PIM context.

Having a route to forming inferential statements is a start, but it does not follow that we can perform *useful* inference for any partially identified model. We need to understand the ramifications of nonidentification—in a given problem, does it render the goal of inferring the target futile? Thus we need to consider the *performance* of Bayesian procedures in partially identified contexts.

Decision-Theoretic Properties

One comforting aspect of the performance of Bayesian procedures derives from the usual decision-theoretic sense in which Bayesian answers are optimal. In brief, consider a loss function which quantifies the "cost" incurred in estimation. In the point-estimation case, for instance, the loss is a function of the true and estimated values of the target; the squared difference between the estimated and true values would be a common choice. We then consider the so-called "Bayes risk" of an estimator—the average loss with respect to the *joint* distribution over parameter and data values, as formed by the prior distribution of parameters and the model distribution of data given parameters. In complete generality, the Bayesian estimator is the estimator which minimizes the Bayes risk. More particularly, the Bayesian estimator or "recipe" is instantiated for a given dataset as the target value minimizing the expected loss with respect to the posterior distribution of parameters given data. Importantly, this sense in which Bayesian procedures are best possible is *completely blind to whether or not the model is identified*. Unlike some of the attractive properties mentioned in Section 1.2, the decision-theoretic optimality of Bayesian procedures is *not* a casualty of nonidentification.

We mentioned correct frequentist interval coverage as a casualty of nonidentification. Still in our camp, however, is a Bayesian sense of correct coverage. Consider an investigator who selects a prior distribution to use for inference, and think of this investigator as playing a "game" against Mother Nature. Specifically, Nature uses a probability distribution to generate the true values of the parameters. In turn, the data are generated given the true values, according to a statistical model. This model, but not the parameter values, is known to the investigator. With respect to this set-up, how well will the investigator's estimation scheme perform? We could ask, for instance, what is the expected loss to be incurred? That is, we could evaluate the Bayes risk with respect to Nature's parameter-generating distribution, for an estimating procedure that takes the investigator's prior distribution as an input.

Bayesian Coverage of Interval Estimators

As described above, if the investigator happens to choose a prior equal to Nature's parameter-generating distribution, then the lowest possible expected loss results. Additionally, in this "nice" situation a calibration property ensues for interval estimation. The investigator can report an interval of target values having a prescribed posterior probability, say 0.95, under the distribution of the target given the observables. More generally, when the prescribed probability is $1 - \alpha$ we call this a $(1 - \alpha)$ credible interval. If the investigator's prior distribution is indeed the same as Nature's parameter-generating distribution, then the chance of the investigator's $(1 - \alpha)$ credible interval containing the true value of the target is indeed $1 - \alpha$. We call this the basic Bayesian calibration of interval estimates, emphasizing that the probability is taken with respect to the joint distribution of parameters and data induced by Nature's choice of distribution for parameters.

Another way to think about this calibration of interval estimates is in terms of an investigator who studies a series of different phenomena in turn. For instance, an epidemiologist might carry out a series of studies of exposure-disease relationships, with one study for each in a series of *different* exposure-disease pairs. An exposure-disease association parameter would be the target of inference in each study. Conceptually, at least, we can think of Nature as using a parameter-generating distribution to disgorge the true parameter values for the sequence of phenomena. Then we can regard coverage in a long-run sense of the proportion of the phenomena for which the corresponding study yields a "good" interval, i.e., containing the true value of the target. If the investigator is able to select a prior distribution matching Nature's parameter-generating distribution, then the investigator is turning out a calibrated product: in 95% of studies undertaken, the 95% interval estimate contains the right answer.

The basic Bayesian calibration for interval estimates has the advantage of relying only on the match between the investigator's prior and Nature's parameter-generating distribution. There are no other caveats. It holds exactly, whether the sample size is small or large, and, most importantly for us, *whether the statistical model is identified or not*. Thus we do have a calibrated way in which to express uncertainty about parameters in the face of partially identified models.

Against this, the proviso that Nature and the investigator share the same distribution over the parameter space is a strong one. Typically, as the two distributions move apart, the calibration will break. And there are good reasons to think that this break can be much worse if the model is not identified. In practice, then, it may be best to think of the calibration in somewhat hypothetical terms: *if* the study at hand were embedded in a sequence of studies for which the true parameter values were drawn from the investigator's prior distribution, *then* the 95% interval estimates would be correct in 95% of these studies.

Another thing to emphasize is that correct Bayesian coverage is indeed a weaker concept than correct frequentist coverage. Say an interval estimation procedure has correct frequentist coverage. Then, for any values of the parameters, the chance of generating a dataset which produces a "good" interval estimate equals the desired coverage. Therefore, averaging this probability across *any* distribution over the parameter space yields the desired coverage, i.e., the Bayesian coverage with respect to any choice of Nature's parameter-generating distribution equals the nominal coverage. Also, importantly, we did not need to know Nature's choice of distribution in order to construct the interval. Thus, all other considerations aside, we would prefer an interval estimator having correct frequentist coverage to one only possessing correct Bayesian coverage. Without model identification, however, correct frequentist coverage is generally impossible to obtain. Therefore, correct Bayesian coverage becomes a fall-back position which can be relied upon in such settings.

1.4   Some Simple Examples of Partially Identified Models

Misclassification of a Binary Variable

Let X be a binary trait of interest, with $X \sim \text{Bernoulli}(p)$ reflecting a prevalence p for trait presence ($X = 1$) rather than absence ($X = 0$), across a population of interest. If independent and identically distributed (*iid*) sampling of X is possible, then estimation of p is a simple matter. The plot thickens somewhat if instead it is only possible to undertake *iid* sampling of X^*, a noisy surrogate for X. For instance, perhaps X^* is obtained from questionnaire self-report, which is not always accurate. Still, if the extent of misclassification is known, one is in good stead. If the *sensitivity* $\gamma_N = Pr(X^* = 1 | X = 1)$ and *specificity* $\gamma_P = Pr(X^* = 0 | X = 0)$ are known quantities, then $X^* \sim \text{Bernoulli}\{(1-r)(1-\gamma_N) + r\gamma_P\}$, and inferring r from an *iid* sample of X^* is still a straightforward exercise in parametric statistical inference.

What if, on the other hand, the extent of misclassification is not completely known? This would likely be the reality, for instance, if X^* arises from self-report on a questionnaire. We then have a game-changer. Clearly inference about r via $\text{Bernoulli}\{(1-r)(1-\gamma_N) + r\gamma_P\}$ observations is not straightforward if (r, γ_N, γ_P) are all unknown. Moreover, while one could easily report inference on the prevalence of X^*, i.e., infer $(1-r)(1-\gamma_N) + r\gamma_P$, this is clearly not the quantity of scientific interest. In fact, one might immediately declare inference on r to be unobtainable, since Bernoulli data can inherently inform only a single parameter (e.g., the prevalence of X^*), whereas three parameters are unknown. Formally, the model indeed lacks identification, since multiple values of the unknown parameters can induce the same distribution of observable data: as an example, consider $(r, \gamma_N, \gamma_P) = (0.2, 0.6, 0.8)$ and $(r, \gamma_N, \gamma_P) = (0.28, 1.0, 1.0)$. Consequently, getting "the right answer," even with an infinite amount of data, is not possible. In Bayesian terms, and in contrast to "textbook" problems, the posterior distribution of r cannot converge to a point-mass at the true value of r as the sample size grows.

In this book, we concede that the right answer cannot be achieved if the data are too limited. In the present example they are doubly limited. First of all, X cannot be measured with complete accuracy. Second, we are not sure of the extent to which the measurements are error-prone. However, we still find it worthwhile to ask questions such as: how well do achievable answers perform, particularly when some background knowledge is available? For instance, say application-area experts are comfortable declaring a worst-case scenario for the extent of misclassification, in the form of lower bounds for each of γ_N and γ_P. Then we would like to know whether this background information, plus a sample of X^*, will likely produce useful inference on the target r. Here, in a big-picture sense, "useful" might be construed as an interval estimate that is narrow enough to justify the cost of collecting the sample. Put another way, perhaps with the aid of background knowledge, we wish to quantify the extent to which limited data can speak to us.

This simple setting of inferring a trait prevalence based on corrupted trait measurements is a launch pad for some more involved problems. One generalization is to multiple populations, e.g., now r_i is the prevalence of X in the i-th population, and differences in prevalence across populations may be of most interest. This is certainly the situation when faced with two particular populations: cases with the disease under study and healthy controls. In this setting X is a binary exposure variable of interest. By a case-control sampling strategy, samples of the error-prone exposure X^* are obtained from each population. An association parameter, such as the ratio of exposure odds for the case population to that of the control population, would be the target of inference. This puts us in the territory of one of the threats-to-validity described in Section 1.1. Moreover, even assuming a simple form for the misclassification process, namely that the sensitivity and specificity are common across populations, we are still in the partially identified world. The two binomial samples can at best fully inform two quantities, yet we are faced with four unknowns: the prevalence of X in each population, along with the sensitivity and specificity of the classification scheme. Another direction in which this problem generalizes is from a binary X and X^* to continuous X and X^*, perhaps in a context where it is suitable to assume some sort of linear error structure, e.g., the surrogate X^* arises as a sum of the actual X plus a "noise" term.

Estimating Properties of Joint Distributions from Marginals

Say that properties of a joint distribution for (X, Y) are of interest, but data on X and Y can only be obtained marginally. As a simple example, say both variables are binary, with $p_{xy} = Pr(X = x, Y = y)$. Disjoint samples of X and Y separately inform $p_{1+} = p_{10} + p_{11} = Pr(X = 1)$ and $p_{+1} = p_{01} + p_{11} = Pr(Y = 1)$, respectively. Consequently, the question of what the data have to say about a joint quantity, p_{11} for instance, can be decomposed as follows: what do the data say directly about (p_{1+}, p_{+1}), and then what is subsequently implied about $(p_{11} | p_{1+}, p_{+1})$ conditionally. The first part of the question is straightforward, since inference about the marginal prevalences is a "textbook" problem in parametric inference. The second part is more subtle, devolving to a conditional distribution arising from whatever joint prior distribution has been specified on the parameters. When we study this problem in the next chapter, we shall see that as with many partially identified problems, a key feature is that the support of the conditional distribution depends on the conditioning arguments. This opens a route for the data to say something about the target.

This problem also has important and interesting generalizations. For instance, a more specialized version of the problem arises in consideration of gene-environment studies. Here aspects of the joint distribution of (Y, X, G) are of interest, where Y is a health outcome, X is an environmental exposure, and G is a genotype. Typically the $(Y | X, G)$ conditional relationship is of most interest. However, sometimes information about (Y, G) comes from a different source than information about X. Thus again the problem is one of inferring a property of a joint distribution from information about its marginals. As we shall see, this problem is nuanced, in that if certain assumptions can be made, the marginals will be more informative about the target. One assumption that is often defensible on the grounds of biologic plausibility is that X and G are independent - the *gene-environment independence* assumption. A further assumption that is defensible in some contexts is that G alone confers no additional risk in the absence of exposure, i.e., $Pr(Y = 1 | X = 0, G = 0) = Pr(Y = 1 | X = 0, G = 1)$. This can be interpreted as saying if G plays a role in the outcome model, it is purely as an effect modifier for X. Once again, the task is to understand information flow. In the face of given background assumptions, to what extent will knowledge about the target be tightened by the accumulation of data?

1.5   The Road Ahead

In the next chapter, we lay out the basic statistical theory and properties surrounding Bayesian inference with a partially identified model. The key idea leveraged is that of *reparameterization*. Particularly, at least some PIMs are amenable to separating out parameters "inside" the likelihood function from those "outside." In turn, those inside are directly informed by observed data, while those outside are at best indirectly informed by data. The chapter describes how reparameterization can assist in computing posterior quantities, and how reparameterization gives insight into properties of Bayesian estimators.

In Chapter 3, the attention turns to an important tradeoff. It is often tempting to make enough background assumptions to achieve model identification, even if one or more of these assumptions is hard to defend. So inference can suffer if we do not make strong assumptions, since only partial identification obtains. But inference can also suffer if we do make strong assumptions, via the general problem that inferences from misspecified models can have poor properties. In this chapter we show that the impact of these deficiencies can be directly compared, one to the other.

Chapters 4, 5 and 6 are devoted to working through some PIM examples in depth. Models for misclassified data are featured in Chapter 4, models involving instrumental variables are featured in Chapter 5, and several further models are considered in Chapter 6. In all instances, the ramifications of partial identification are examined, particularly in terms of how inferences change, and particularly the extent to which they sharpen or not, as more data accumulate.

Then in Chapter 7 we discuss some further topics and future research directions. After some brief remarks on computational issues, the emphasis shifts to characterizing the value of information obtained from data in a partially identified context. This speaks to the question of how much data is worth collecting. Also in Chapter 7, we review some of the real-data applications of PIMs that have recently appeared in the literature. We close in Chapter 8 with some final thoughts on the past and present state of affairs with partial identification.

Chapter 2

The Structure of Inference in Partially Identified Models

2.1 Bayesian Inference

Bayes Theorem

Say that a scientific problem presents itself in the form of n datapoints d_n linked to a vector of unknown parameters θ according to a statistical model, with this model expressed in the form of a conditional density function $\pi(d_n|\theta)$. Moreover, inferences will be relative to a proper prior distribution for the parameters, expressed as a marginal density function $\pi(\theta)$. In committing to a choice of prior distribution and a choice of statistical model, the analyst has defined a joint distribution of observables and unobservables, to wit $\pi(\theta, d_n) = \pi(\theta)\pi(d_n|\theta)$. Bayes theorem, which simply corresponds to deducing the conditional distribution of the parameters given the data, is expressed as

$$\pi(\theta|d_n) = \frac{\pi(d_n|\theta)\pi(\theta)}{\int \pi\left(d_n|\tilde{\theta}\right)\pi\left(\tilde{\theta}\right)d\tilde{\theta}}. \tag{2.1}$$

Under the Bayesian paradigm, (2.1) characterizes knowledge about the parameter values having observed the data values. We assume the reader has some basic exposure to Bayesian analysis, so that (2.1) can be used without much further ado. If this is not the case, the reader is recommended to consult one of the now numerous books that introduce the Bayesian approach (suggestions include Bolstad, 2007; Hoff, 2009; Carlin and Louis, 2011; Christensen et al., 2011; Lee, 2012; Gelman et al., 2013) .

Notation

Before focusing on identification issues, we set some notational conventions for the rest of the book. By discussing this now we endure some short-term pain for the sake of long-term gain. While often glossed over, exposition of Bayesian material can present a notational nightmare. In the statistical literature generally, it is absolutely standard to use Greek letters for unknown parameters that must be estimated from data. Hence the θ in (2.1), for instance.

Unfortunately, though, the Bayesian literature is rife with exposition where the meaning of θ shifts back and forth subtly. For instance, on the same page one could see:

- The use of θ as one or more parameters in generic terms, so that expressions like "θ is the population odds-ratio measuring association between the two binary traits" makes sense, and use of θ as in (2.1) is acceptable.

- The use of θ as a random variable, so we can legitimately write mathematical expressions for moments and probabilities associated with prior and posterior quantities. Hence phrasings such as $Pr(\theta < 0.5) = 0.34$, or $E(\theta|d_n) = 0.73$ are coherent.

- The use of θ as the true but unknown value of a parameter, so we can say things like " as the data accumulate, the posterior distribution converges to a point mass at θ."

Even though we will not insist on much mathematical rigor in this book, using the same symbol in all three of these roles is clearly uncomfortable.

Perhaps some clarity is gained via the usual probabilistic convention that uppercase and lowercase letters distinguish between random variables and their instantiated values, respectively. For instance, it seems like progress to pen statements such as: "the posterior mean $E(\Theta|d_n)$ estimates the parameter θ." However, here we are hampered because many of us do not associate the lowercase and uppercase versions of some Greek letters as quickly and innately as we do for Latin letters. For instance, writing "events" as $\{\Lambda = \lambda\}$ or $\{\Sigma = \sigma\}$ is just not as natural to the reader as $\{A = a\}$ or $\{B = b\}$. And to make matters worse, another overwhelmingly adopted convention in the statistical literature is to use uppercase counterparts to denote parameter spaces. We cannot seriously write a posterior mean as $E(\Theta \mid d_n)$ if we earlier wrote $\theta \in \Theta$ to denote all the possible values the parameter could take on.

This Greek tragicomedy of notation does not hamper the exposition of frequentist statistical ideas, where distributions are never applied to parameters. But thinking about distributions on parameters is the lifeblood of Bayesian statistics. We must be able to move back and forth seamlessly between a parameter as a fixed but unknown quantity and a probability distribution which quantifies our knowledge about this quantity. So, we try something completely different. We still use lowercase Greek letters, like θ, to represent one or all the unknown parameters in a statistical model. However, when our Bayesian purpose *absolutely demands* a corresponding random variable, in particular inside mathematical operators like $E()$ and $Pr()$, we will denote this using a "star" superscript. That is $\theta^\star$ is a random variable marginally distributed according to the assigned prior distribution with density function $\pi(\theta)$. And, for instance, the posterior mean of θ is expressed as $E(\theta^\star \mid d_n)$, or perhaps $E(\theta^\star|d_n^\star = d_n)$.

Similarly, we want a notation that can easily emphasize the true values of one or more parameters when needed. Some authors use a "nought" subscript for this purpose. If θ is a vector of parameters, however, then θ_0 could possibly be confused for one element of θ rather than the true value of the whole vector. Thus we instead reserve the use of a "dagger" superscript to indicate the true value of a parameter vector under which the observable data are spawned. Thus a phrase like "we can estimate θ by $E(\theta^\star|d_n)$, which converges to $\theta^\dagger$ as n increases" is fair game, at least as far as this book is concerned.

The other notational quandary we face involves the expression of density functions. In fact we have already abused notation by using $\pi()$ to represent different things, depending on the argument supplied. For instance, with respect to the joint distribution induced by the model and prior specifications we write $\pi(\theta)$ for the prior density, $\pi(d_n|\theta)$ for the model density, $\pi(d_n) = \int \pi(d_n|\theta)\pi(\theta)d\theta$ for the marginal density of the data, and so on. A more formal notation might involve a subscript on $\pi()$ to indicate *which* density we are talking about; however, this notation quickly becomes overwhelming. So we ask for the reader's indulgence in letting the argument supplied to $\pi()$ signal which $\pi()$ we are talking about. Admittedly this is a loose notation, particularly as we make much use of reparameterizations in this book. So we might see statements like $\omega = h(\theta)$ for an invertible function $h()$, hence

$$\pi(\omega) \quad = \quad \pi(h^{-1}(\omega))\left|(h^{-1})'(\omega)\right|,$$

or simply

$$\pi(\omega) \quad = \quad \pi(\theta(\omega))\left|\frac{\partial\theta}{\partial\omega}\right|.$$

Please take such equations in the spirit intended!

2.2   The Structure of Posterior Distributions in Partially Identified Models

Transparent Reparameterizations

As stated in Chapter 1, a statistical model lacks identification if multiple values of the parameter vector correspond to the same distribution of observables. Put more positively, a model possesses identification if $\pi(d_n|\theta^{(1)}) = \pi(d_n|\theta^{(2)})$ implies that $\theta^{(1)} = \theta^{(2)}$. There is, of course, a vast literature on varied aspects surrounding Bayesian updating as per (2.1). However, the subset of this literature looking at situations where the statistical model $\pi(d_n|\theta)$ lacks identification is rather small (see, for instance, Kadane, 1974; Dawid, 1979; Neath and Samaniego, 1997; Poirier, 1998; Gustafson, 2005a). In this chapter we take quite a general look at the behavior of the posterior $\pi(\theta|d_n)$ in the face of "partial" identification. Temporarily, however, we will be coy about the precise meaning of partial.

At least initially, the statistical model at hand is assumed to be expressed in terms that are scientifically meaningful. By this we mean that to the extent possible, the components of θ have interpretations that are accessible and meaningful to subject-area scientists. This should help such experts in the elicitation process of choosing a proper prior distribution with density $\pi(\theta)$. Once the model is specified and the prior chosen, however, the choice of parameterization is mathematically arbitrary: it simply provides a "coordinate system" in which to determine posterior quantities. If $h()$ is a smooth, invertible function, then Bayesian inference could equally well be carried out in terms of $\tilde{\theta} = h(\theta)$ rather than θ.

While ultimately the answers obtained do not depend on the choice of parameterization under which they are computed, some parameterizations can lend more intuition about the flow of information in a partially identified model context. Sometimes it is possible to move from the original, "scientific" parameterization to a new parameterization with particular properties that shed light on the efficacy of inference.

For a model lacking identification, say it is possible to reparameterize according to $(\phi, \lambda) = h(\theta)$ such that two properties hold:

(i) The distribution of the data depends only on ϕ, not on λ, i.e., $\pi(d_n | \phi, \lambda) = \pi(d_n | \phi)$.

(ii) Regular parametric asymptotic theory applies to the model $\pi(d_n | \phi)$, so that $\sqrt{n}$ consistent estimation of ϕ obtains.

Then (ϕ, λ) is referred to as a **transparent reparameterization**. Necessarily, of course, $\dim(\phi) + \dim(\lambda) = \dim(\theta)$.

It is worth noting that transparent parameterizations are not unique, and particularly the choice of λ is usually rather arbitrary. That is, all sorts of functions of θ having $\dim(\theta) - \dim(\phi)$ components could do the job. Generally though, if $(\phi^{(1)}, \lambda^{(1)})$ and $(\phi^{(2)}, \lambda^{(2)})$ are both transparent parameterizations, then the map from $\phi^{(1)}$ to $\phi^{(2)}$ will be invertible. That is, there cannot be ambiguity about what quantities influence the distribution of the data. Also note that condition (ii) is important. It effectively means that the dimension of ϕ is as small as possible whilst satisfying (i). That is, ϕ cannot carry redundant components which do not actually impact the distribution of the observable data. In the terminology of Barankin (1960), ϕ is a *minimal sufficient* parameter.

If a transparent parameterization can be found, then it does lay bare the flow of information, since

$$\pi(\phi, \lambda | d_n) = \frac{\pi(d_n | \phi, \lambda) \pi(\phi, \lambda)}{\pi(d_n)}$$

$$= \frac{\pi(d_n | \phi) \pi(\phi)}{\pi(d_n)} \pi(\lambda | \phi)$$

$$= \pi(\phi | d_n) \pi(\lambda | \phi).$$

So the posterior marginal distribution of ϕ is based on "standard" updating, starting from the prior marginal distribution of ϕ. However, the posterior conditional distribution of $(\lambda | \phi)$ is the same as the prior conditional distribution, regardless of the quantity or nature of the data.

We tacitly assume that the specified prior distribution for θ induces a nicely behaved $\pi(\phi)$. This, in tandem with the regular asymptotic behavior of the model $\pi(d_n | \phi)$, leads to "textbook" behavior of the posterior marginal distribution $\pi(\phi | d_n)$. By this we mean concentration to a single point as the data accumulate. Moreover, assuming the statistical model is correctly specified, this single point will be the right point, i.e., $\pi(\phi | d_n)$ will tend to a point mass at $\phi^\dagger$. Thus the situation as the sample size increases is governed by a very simple characterization.

In the limit of an infinite amount of data, the posterior distribution of the parameters is described by a point mass at $\phi = \phi^\dagger$ combined with the conditional prior distribution $\pi(\lambda | \phi^\star = \phi^\dagger)$. Henceforth this is referred to as the **limiting posterior distribution** (LPD).

The above statement emphasizes clarity over rigor. As already suggested, the statistical model and prior for (d_n, ϕ) are presumed to be sufficiently smooth and well-behaved such that standard asymptotic arguments apply. A more formal statement of the limiting behavior would be that for any neighborhood A of $\phi^\dagger$, the random variable $B_n = Pr\{\phi \in A | d_n^\star\}$ converges almost surely to one as n increases. One key condition needed for this is that the data d_n indeed arise as independent and identically distributed draws from the postulated model distribution with $\phi = \phi^\dagger$. For more on both the concepts of Bayesian asymptotics and the requisite regularity conditions, see, for instance, the review of Ghosal (1996).

Very often a single parameter is of most inferential interest. With respect to the initial parameterization, we shall denote a scalar parameter of interest or *target of inference* as $\psi - \tilde{g}(\theta)$. And when we move to a transparent parameterization we express this same target as $\psi = g(\phi, \lambda)$, i.e., $g() = \tilde{g}\{h^{-1}()\}$. Consequently, the LPD on the target is the distribution of $g(\phi^\dagger, \lambda)$ that is induced by the prior conditional distribution $\pi(\lambda | \phi^\star = \phi^\dagger)$.

In this book we are most interested in situations where $g()$ varies non-trivially with respect to both its arguments. Then, roughly speaking, the LPD on the target will be (i), more spread out than a point mass distribution at the true value $\psi^{\dagger} = g(\phi^{\dagger}, \lambda^{\dagger})$, but (ii), more concentrated than the prior distribution of $\psi = g(\phi, \lambda)$. This "intermediate" nature of the posterior distribution on the target, even after observing an infinite amount of data, embodies the *partial* information often available in partially identified modelling contexts.

Strength of Bayesian Updating

With a transparent reparameterization at hand, there is a qualitative spectrum for the extent to which observable data inform the target parameter of interest. Perfect learning will arise only if the target ψ is a function of ϕ alone, in which case we might say the target parameter is fully identified. On the other hand, a perfect *absence* of learning, whereby the LPD and prior for ψ are the same, requires that (i), the target is a function of λ alone, and (ii), ϕ and λ are independent *a priori*. When this happens we might say the target is fully unidentified.

In between these two extremes, the situation is further delineated by the nature of the prior dependence between ϕ and λ. Remember that the prior distribution is initially supplied in the scientifically meaningful parameterization θ, with elicitation judgments about *a priori* dependencies made in this frame of reference. It becomes important to see what dependence structure is then induced in terms of (ϕ, λ). Special attention is given to the *support* of the conditional density, i.e., given a value of ϕ, for what values of λ is $\pi(\lambda|\phi) > 0$? For the sake of clarity going forward, we create some terms to describe the prior dependence between ϕ and λ.

With respect to a given choice of prior $\pi(\theta)$, a transparent reparameterization from θ to (ϕ, λ) is described as:

- **factorable**, if ϕ and λ are independent under π;
- **loose**, if ϕ and λ are dependent under π, but the support of $\pi(\lambda \mid \phi)$ does not vary with ϕ, and consequently is the same as the support of $\pi(\lambda)$;

- **sticky**, if ϕ and λ are dependent under π and the support of $\pi(\lambda|\phi)$ varies with ϕ, so that the support of $\pi(\lambda|\phi)$ is a proper subset of the support of $\pi(\lambda)$, at least for some values of ϕ.

When working on a partially identified problem with a particular choice of prior, it is important to be aware whether the chosen transparent parameterization is factorable, loose, or sticky. Having said that though, it is also important to note that this does not characterize the problem itself. For instance, say that $\dim(\lambda) = 1$, and for the given prior π, (ϕ, λ) constitutes a sticky transparent parameterization. Particularly, say the support of $\pi(\lambda|\phi)$ is an interval with endpoints depending on ϕ, say $(a(\phi), b(\phi))$. Upon taking $\tilde{\lambda} = \{\lambda - a(\phi)\}/\{b(\phi) - a(\phi)\}$, $(\phi, \tilde{\lambda})$ would constitute a loose transparent parameterization of the same problem. A more definitive characterization arises from consideration of the prior dependence between ϕ and the target of inference.

With respect to a given choice of prior $\pi(\theta)$ and an arbitrary transparent parameterization (ϕ, λ), say $\psi = g(\phi, \lambda)$ is the scalar target of inference. We say there is:

• **no indirect learning** about ψ, if ψ and ϕ are independent under π;

• **weak indirect learning** about ψ, if ψ and ϕ are dependent under π, but the support of $\pi(\psi|\phi)$ does not vary with ϕ, and consequently is the same as the support of $\pi(\psi)$;

• **strong indirect learning** about ψ, if ψ and ϕ are dependent under π and the support of $\pi(\psi|\phi)$ varies with ϕ. Consequently, the support of $\pi(\psi|\phi)$ is a proper subset of the support of $\pi(\psi)$, for at least some values of ϕ.

The notion of strong indirect learning dovetails with the literature on partial identification and parameter bounds, as described, for instance, by Manski (2003). Only a subset of the *a priori* possible values of the target may cohere with the law of the observable data, with this law being revealed to the analyst in the limit of an infinite sample size. Thus the *identification region* for the target spoken of in non-Bayesian approaches to partial identification is identically the support of the LPD for the target, which, in turn, is equivalently the support of the conditional prior distribution $\pi(\psi|\phi^{\dagger})$.

Conceptually, if an infinitely large dataset were actually available, the non-Bayesian statistician could simply report the identification region for the target parameter as "the result" of an analysis. In contrast, a Bayesian statistician would be inclined, if not beholden, to report the limiting posterior distribution over the identification region as the fundamental result. Note that this distinction is much stronger in the face of partial identification than it is for full identification. For a fully identified target, the large-sample limit of its posterior distribution is a point mass and its identification region tends to the corresponding point.

Returning to reality at least momentarily, of course an infinite-sized dataset is purely fictional. With a real dataset a Bayesian would view the posterior distribution over the target parameter as the fundamental output of an analysis. The LPD is still relevant though, since

$$
\begin{aligned}
\pi(\psi|d_n) &= \int \pi(\psi|\phi,d_n)\pi(\phi|d_n)d\phi \\
&= \int \pi(\psi|\phi)\pi(\phi|d_n)d\phi,
\end{aligned}
\tag{2.2}
$$

i.e., the finite-sample posterior over the target is a mixture of LPDs arising from different values of ϕ, weighted according to the posterior marginal distribution of ϕ. Particularly, in the case of strong indirect learning we can intuit that (2.2) induces a "fuzzy" identification region by mixing across $\pi(\psi|\phi)$ having differing support. A non-Bayesian has different options. For instance, in the $\dim(\lambda) = 1$ case with the identification region being an interval, point estimation of both interval endpoints would be a place to start.

Example A: Inferring Joint Properties from Marginal Distributions

Here we pick up in earnest on the problem mentioned in Section 1.4, where the task is to infer properties of a joint distribution from data on marginals. Recall that the population distribution of a pair of binary variables (X,Y) is initially parameterized as $p_{xy} = Pr(X = x, Y = y)$, so the scientific parameterization can be taken to be $\theta = (p_{01}, p_{10}, p_{11})$ (with p_{00} implicitly being one minus the sum of these three probabilities). Prior beliefs could be captured with a Dirichlet prior distribution, i.e.,

$$
\pi(p_{01}, p_{10}, p_{11}) \propto (1 - p_{01} - p_{10} - p_{11})^{c_{00}-1} p_{01}^{c_{01}-1} p_{10}^{c_{10}-1} p_{11}^{c_{11}-1} \times
$$
$$
I\{\min(p_{01}, p_{10}, p_{11}) > 0, p_{01} + p_{10} + p_{11} < 1\} \tag{2.3}
$$

for chosen positive hyperparameters $c_{\bullet\bullet} = (c_{00}, c_{01}, c_{10}, c_{11})$. The observable data are presumed to arise via an *iid* sample of size n_x in which only X can be measured, with t_x out of n_x subjects having $X = 1$. Independently of this, an *iid* sample of size n_y in which only Y can be measured leads to t_y of n_y subjects having $Y = 1$. Such a study design could arise, for instance, if privacy provisions rule out acquisition of both X and Y for the same subject. Clearly the resulting likelihood function is based on $t_x^* \sim \text{Binomial}(n_x, p_{10} + p_{11})$ and independently $t_y^* \sim \text{Binomial}(n_y, p_{01} + p_{11})$.

A sticky transparent parameterization for this problem is obtained as $\phi = (q, r)$, $\lambda = s$, where $q = p_{10} + p_{11} = Pr(X = 1)$, $r = p_{01} + p_{11} = Pr(Y = 1)$, $s = p_{11} = Pr(X = 1, Y = 1)$. Transforming (2.3) in this instance is particularly straightforward, since the map $h()$ from θ to (ϕ, λ) is linear. Specifically, we obtain:

$$
\pi(q, r, s) \propto (1 - q - r + s)^{c_{00}-1}(r - s)^{c_{01}-1}(q - s)^{c_{10}-1}s^{c_{11}-1} \times
$$

$$I\{0 < q < 1, 0 < r < 1\} \times$$
$$I\{\max(0, q + r - 1) < s < \min(q, r)\}. \tag{2.4}$$

Then joint inference on (q, r, s) arises upon multiplying (2.4) by the likelihood $q^{t_x}(1 - q)^{n_x - t_x} r^{t_y}(1 - r)^{n_y - t_y}$, to obtain the posterior density $\pi(q, r, s | t_x, t_y)$, at least up to a constant of proportionality.

As the sample sizes n_x and n_y increase, $\pi(q, r | t_x, t_y)$ will tend to a point mass at the true values $(q^\dagger, r^\dagger)$. On the other hand, the absence of s from the likelihood function immediately implies $\pi(s | q, r, t_x, t_y) = \pi(s | q, r)$. Thus, as the sample sizes grow, the limiting marginal posterior density on s will be $\pi(s | q^\dagger, r^\dagger)$, the conditional prior distribution with conditioning on the correct values of (q, r). The form of this conditional density is immediately "read off" from (2.4), by regarding this expression as a function of s for fixed (q, r). So the limiting distribution has density

$$\pi(s \mid q^\dagger, r^\dagger) \quad \propto \quad (1 - q^\dagger - r^\dagger + s)^{c_{00}-1}(r^\dagger - s)^{c_{01}-1} \times$$
$$(q^\dagger - s)^{c_{10}-1} s^{c_{11}-1} \times$$
$$I\{\max(0, q^\dagger + r^\dagger - 1) < s < \min(q^\dagger, r^\dagger)\}. \tag{2.5}$$

A number of things can and should be noted about (2.5). First, the interval $(\max\{0, q^\dagger + r^\dagger - 1\}, \min\{q^\dagger, r^\dagger\})$ is the identification region for the target parameter $s = p_{11}$. This interval, comprising all the values of the target compatible with the observed data, is revealed to the analyst upon obtaining an infinite number of observations, i.e., upon learning $q = q^\dagger, r = r^\dagger$. The particular form of the identification region for this problem is unsurprising: the bounds are particular instances of the Fréchet inequalities for the probability of a conjunction (Fréchet, 1951). Second, a special case of interest is $(c_{00}, c_{01}, c_{10}, c_{11}) = (1, 1, 1, 1)$, corresponding to a uniform prior distribution over the (X, Y) cell probabilities. In this case the LPD (2.5) devolves to a uniform distribution over the identification region, with no parameter values inside the region favored over any others.

The plot thickens when non-uniform priors on θ are selected. Consider, for instance, the hyperparameter choice $(c_{00}, c_{01}, c_{10}, c_{11}) = (2, 2, 2, 2)$. This downweights very small and large cell probabilities, and can be interpreted as a prior with an "effective sample size" of eight data observations. Marginally it implies $p_{xy} \sim \text{Beta}(2, 6)$ *a priori*, for $x, y = 0, 1$. Figure 2.1 portrays the resulting LPD for the target parameter $s = p_{11}$, for four different values of the true marginal probabilities $(q^\dagger, r^\dagger)$. Note that the first two cases, $(q^\dagger, r^\dagger) = (0.2, 0.2)$ and $(q^\dagger, r^\dagger) = (0.2, 0.75)$, give rise to the *same* identification region but *different* limiting posterior densities over this region. More generally, this can happen when $q^\dagger + r^\dagger \leq 1$, since in this case the identification region is the interval from zero to $\min(q^\dagger, r^\dagger)$, but the shape of the density depends on both $\min(q^\dagger, r^\dagger)$ and $\max(q^\dagger, r^\dagger)$. Thus in some circumstances the data have an ability to speak that goes beyond determining the identification region and then having the shape of the LPD over this region follow automatically.

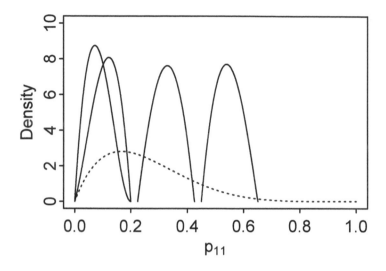

Figure 2.1 *Four limiting posterior densities for $p_{11} = Pr(X = 1, Y = 1)$ in Example A, with a Dirichlet(2,2,2,2) prior on p_{xy}. From left to right, X and Y have marginal prevalences of $(0.2, 0.2)$, $(0.2, 0.75)$, $(0.425, 0.8)$, and $(0.65, 0.8)$. All these settings induce an identification interval with width 0.2. The dotted curve is the Beta(2,6) prior marginal density for the target.*

On the other hand, when $q^{\dagger} + r^{\dagger} > 1$, the identification interval runs from $q^{\dagger} + r^{\dagger} - 1$ to $\min\{q^{\dagger}, r^{\dagger}\}$). In this case there is a one-to-one relationship between the endpoints of the identification region and the shape of the limiting posterior density. In such a case the data have less to say beyond the determination of the identification region - though the shape of the LPD still points out that some values in the region are *a posteriori* more plausible than others. Also, note that the shape is not trivially predicted from the chosen prior distribution without actually determining the LPD. Particularly, Figure 2.1 reveals that in cases where $q^{\dagger} + r^{\dagger} > 1$, the unimodal shape of the LPD is quite different than the shape of the prior density truncated to the identification region. In comparing the plausibility of two different values inside the identification region, there can be substantial prior-to-posterior updating. Some of these ideas about separating out the information in the data about the whereabouts of the identification region from the further information about the shape of the posterior distribution over this region are taken up later in this chapter. ■

2.3 Computational Strategies

Computing Limiting Posterior Distributions

The strategy used to determine the LPD in Example A can in fact be expressed in very general terms, and applied in a wide array of problems. Recall that the transparent reparameterization takes the form $(\phi, \lambda) = h(\theta)$ for an invertible function $h()$. We presume that computer functions can be written to evaluate both $h()$ and $h^{-1}()$ at arbitrary input values. In some cases a closed-form expression for $h^{-1}()$ may be obtained, while in others, numerical methods may be required. Either way, as a sanity check it should be verified that the coded functions are indeed inverses of each other, at a suite of test points.

Similarly, code to evaluate $h'()$ and $(h^{-1})'()$ must be written. In situations where $h^{-1}()$ has a closed-form, then both $h'()$ and $(h^{-1})'()$ can be based on analytic expressions, and for a suite of test points it should be verified that $|(h^{-1})'()| = |h'(h^{-1}())|^{-1}$ is indeed obtained. In cases where $h^{-1}()$ can only be evaluated numerically, it will instead be necessary to take this identity as a route to evaluating $|(h^{-1})'()|$ via evaluation of $|h'()|$, hence an empirical test on the coding is not available. In any event, once armed with code that is tested as much as possible, the limiting posterior distribution arising for true parameter values $\theta^\dagger$ can be determined numerically as follows.

Consider the case that $\dim(\lambda) = 1$. Given code to evaluate $\pi(\theta)$, $h(\theta)$, $h^{-1}(\phi, \lambda)$, and $|(h^{-1})'(\phi, \lambda)|$, the LPD arising when $\theta = \theta^\dagger$ can be computed by the following steps.

1. Evaluate $(\phi^\dagger, \lambda^\dagger) = h(\theta^\dagger)$.

2. For a grid of points $\lambda^{(1)} < \lambda^{(2)} < \ldots < \lambda^{(m)}$ evaluate the prior conditional density $\pi(\lambda | \phi^\dagger)$ up to a normalizing constant via

$$\pi(\lambda^{(j)} | \phi^\dagger) \quad \propto \quad \pi(h^{-1}(\phi^\dagger, \lambda^{(j)})) \left| (h^{-1})'(\phi^\dagger, \lambda^{(j)}) \right|.$$

3. Use an appropriate numerical integration scheme to normalize, and thereby obtain a grid-defined numerical representation of $\pi(\lambda | \phi^\dagger)$. Any limiting posterior quantities of interest can be expressed as quantities associated with this distribution.

Some remarks about this algorithm are in order. First, when $\dim(\lambda) > 1$, the generalization to a higher-dimensional grid of λ values is readily apparent. Second, in problems where the support of $\pi(\lambda | \phi)$ can be determined in closed-form, the chosen gridpoints in step 2 need only cover this support. Failing this, the gridpoints can be chosen to cover the marginal prior support of $\pi(\lambda)$, then $\pi(\lambda^{(j)}|\phi^\dagger)$ will be computed as being zero or positive for each j, as appropriate. Finally, note that the algorithm described is completely dependent on being able to find a transparent parameterization. However, there is some work in the literature on the much harder situation of a partially identified model for which a transparent parameterization is not easily found (Gustafson, 2009; Jones et al., 2010).

Computing Posterior Distributions

Returning briefly to Figure 2.1, note that two extremes are being compared: a prior distribution describing knowledge about the target parameter in the absence of any data, and a limiting posterior distribution showing the updating of knowledge upon receiving an infinite amount of data. In between these extremes lies the reality of having some data. Toward presenting some examples of finite-sample inference in partially identified models, we need some discussion of Bayesian inference. For a given model $\pi(d_n|\theta)$ and prior $\pi(\theta)$, the usual array of computational options for Bayesian inference presents itself.

An applications-oriented user who wishes to shield himself from implementation issues might consider general-purpose software to implement Markov Chain Monte Carlo (MCMC) algorithms. Such software takes model and prior specifications as inputs, and provides a Monte Carlo sample from the posterior distribution as output. Various versions of the BUGS software, particulary WinBUGS (Lunn et al., 2000) are long-standing and widely used in this regard. And a much newer entrant, Stan (Stan Development Team, 2013), seems promising.

General-purpose software has facilitated an enormous amount of applied Bayesian statistical work. Without full identification, however, the situation can be problematic. A typical Bayesian application of a partially identified model might involve a prior distribution constructed from "standard" distributions in the original θ parameterization (in which the components of θ are scientifically meaningful). But, as we have already seen, a standard prior distribution in the θ parameterization can induce a highly non-standard prior distribution in the (ϕ, λ) parameterization. Consequently, general-purpose Bayesian software cannot be applied in the (ϕ, λ) parameterization, since the non-standard prior distribution is not supported by the software. So, the use of general-purpose software is likely limited to the θ parameterization.

General-purpose software will attempt to use typical MCMC computational algorithms *in the parameterization provided.* For instance, the software may attempt one-by-one updates to the univariate components of θ, perhaps using Gibbs sampling (Gelfand and Smith, 1990) when possible, and random walk Metropolis-Hastings updates (Hastings, 1970; Tierney, 1994) when not possible. Unfortunately such a scheme will often work very poorly in partially identified contexts, precisely because of the lack of identification. Roughly put, "ridges" and "flat spots" in the likelihood function for θ will tend to trip up component-by-component updating of θ, in a way that is much more perverse than for identified models.

In light of this, at least for problems where the number of parameters is modest and a transparent parameterization can be found, we will consider a computational strategy that acknowledges the lack of model identification. As a first thought, we might consider applying standard computational approaches to the embedded identified model $\pi(d_n|\phi)$ and the corresponding marginal prior $\pi(\phi)$. That is, we might attempt to divide our computational task into going after the posterior marginal $\pi(\phi|d_n)$ and the prior conditional $\pi(\lambda|\phi)$, since these characterize the joint posterior distribution. However, as alluded to above, we may not even have a closed-form expression for the marginal prior density $\pi(\phi)$. This precludes the application of standard MCMC techniques to compute $\pi(\phi|d_n)$.

What we do have going for us, however, is that regular asymptotic behavior applies to $\pi(d_n|\phi)$. Hence it may be easy to go after the posterior on ϕ that arises under a wrong, but convenient, choice of prior distribution on ϕ. If we also commit to a wrong yet convenient choice of prior distribution for λ given ϕ, then we can put forth a fairly general strategy based on *importance sampling*.

Say that we have a transparent parameterization such that the joint prior density $\pi(\phi, \lambda)$ can be evaluated. Choose a convenience prior density $\pi^*(\phi, \lambda)$ by specifying the marginal density $\pi^*(\phi)$ and the conditional density $\pi^*(\lambda|\phi)$.

Step 1. Simulate a Monte Carlo sample of size m from the posterior distribution arising from the convenience prior, i.e., a sample from $\pi^*(\phi, \lambda|d_n) = \pi^*(\phi|d_n)\pi^*(\lambda|\phi)$. Denote this sample as $(\phi^{(i)}, \lambda^{(i)})$, $i = 1, \ldots, m$.

Step 2. Compute importance weights with

$$w_i \quad \propto \quad \frac{\pi\left(\phi^{(i)}, \lambda^{(i)}\right)}{\pi^*\left(\phi^{(i)}\right)\pi^*\left(\lambda^{(i)}|\phi^{(i)}\right)}, \qquad (2.6)$$

scaled such that $\sum_{i=1}^{m} w_i = 1$.

Then the weighted version of the generated sample represents the desired posterior distribution $\pi(\phi, \lambda|d_n)$.

Quite a few things should be noted here. The overarching point is that we are representing the joint posterior density proportional to $\pi(d_n|\phi)\pi(\phi,\lambda)$ using Monte Carlo realizations from the "wrong" joint posterior density proportional to $\pi(d_n|\phi)\pi^*(\phi,\lambda)$, by assigning weights to the simulated values. And because both the sampled distribution and target distribution are posterior distributions arising via the same likelihood function for ϕ, the likelihood contributions cancel in the numerator and denominator of the weights. Thus the expression for w_i is free of the data d_n, and the only variation in the weights arises from differences between the convenience and actual prior densities. In many situations this variation is modest, hence the computation is efficient.

As some more specific comments, first, it may be possible to both (i), choose $\pi^*(\phi)$ to be conjugate prior for the "embedded" identified model $\pi(d_n|\phi)$, and (ii), choose $\pi^*(\lambda|\phi)$ to be a standard distribution. Then direct *iid* sampling will be possible in Step 1, rather than MCMC sampling. This constitutes a considerable simplification.

Second, if the parameterization is sticky, then the support of $\pi^*(\lambda|\phi)$ must contain the support of $\pi(\lambda|\phi)$, for every ϕ, in order for the algorithm to be valid. However, having the support of $\pi^*(\lambda|\phi)$ be unnecessarily larger than the support of $\pi(\lambda|\phi)$ will be inefficient, as draws falling outside the smaller support will be assigned zero weight. Ideally, then, the convenience prior conditional distribution can be chosen such that its support is the same as the actual prior conditional distribution.

Third, as usual with importance sampling, it is not necessary to keep track of multiplicative constants in the weight calculation. Note, however, that any multiplicative terms in $\pi^*(\lambda|\phi)$ that depends on ϕ are *not* constant in the expression for $\pi^*(\phi,\lambda)$, so these must be retained in the calculation.

Finally, a nice general feature of importance sampling is that the worth of weighted sample can be summarized by the *effective sample size, ESS =* $1/(\sum_{i=1}^m w_i^2)$ (Doucet et al., 2001). In situations where Step 1 can be realized via *iid* sampling, this has a particularly nice interpretation: in terms of representing the target distribution, the weighted sample of m points carries as much information as an *iid* sample of $ESS < m$ points.

Aside: What to Do with Monte Carlo Output?

Bayesian analysis is very often implemented via some form of Monte Carlo sampling of the posterior distribution. And commonly one wishes to "see" univariate marginal posterior distributions, perhaps before moving on to report more formal posterior quantities, such as moments or quantiles. A histogram and a kernel density estimate are two standard tools for visualizing a univariate distribution based only on a sample of values drawn from that distribution. Of course, both these tools require some input concerning *smoothing*, via the choice of bins for a histogram, or the choice of bandwidth for a density estimate.

As a convention for this book, we will use histograms rather than kernel density estimates. While density estimates are generally more realistic in their smoothness, they are known to struggle around "edges" of datasets. And, particularly when using Monte Carlo sampling to represent LPDs, we can encounter unusually abrupt edges: sampled values pile up on one side of an identification interval boundary, but not the other. So, while histograms are unrealistically "boxy," we prefer them. Indeed, their boxy nature serves to remind us that recovering a smooth density function from even a large Monte Carlo sample is a challenging endeavor.

Having committed to histograms to represent posterior marginal distributions when Monte Carlo techniques are employed, we still have some implementation choices. This is particularly the case when importance sampling is the Monte Carlo scheme in question. Clearly we cannot simply plot bin frequencies when points in some bins carry more weight than others. Fortunately, several R packages provide the facility to generate a "weighted histogram" (Lumley, 2004; Pasek et al., 2012). Or, a quick fix is to resample the Monte Carlo sample in a weighted manner, so that bin frequencies for the new sample do indeed reflect the distribution of interest. Then standard software to generate a histogram can be applied. To avoid introducing unnecessary further Monte Carlo variation, however, the new sample should be very large. Indeed, it is fine to make it larger than the original sample.

Presuming that equally wide bins are used in the histogram construction, a final issue is the choice of how many bins. Many software routines use the suggestion dating back to Sturges (1926), of using $\lceil \log_2 m + 1 \rceil$ bins for a sample of m points. However, bearing in mind that a weighted sample of m points carries less information than an *iid* sample of m points, when using importance sampling we modify this guidance to $\lceil \log_2 ESS + 1 \rceil$ bins. ★

Example A, Continued

To compute the posterior distribution arising from a finite sample in this problem, we can take $\pi^*(q, r)$ to be the uniform distribution on $(0, 1) \times (0, 1)$ and $\pi^*(s|q, r)$ to the uniform distribution on the identification interval $(\min\{q, r\}, \max\{0 + q + r - 1\})$. It follows immediately that $\pi^*(q, r|t_x, t_y) = \pi^*(q|t_x)\pi^*(r|t_y)$ is characterized by the Beta$(1 + t_x, 1 + n_x - t_x)$ and Beta$(1 + t_y, 1 + n_y - t_y)$ distributions, respectively. Hence *iid* sampling from $\pi^*(q, r, s|t_x, t_y) = \pi^*(q, r|t_x, t_y)\pi^*(s|q, r)$ is easily implemented. And the importance weights (2.6) take the form $w_i - w(q^{(i)}, r^{(i)}, s^{(i)})$, where

$$w(q, r, s) \propto (1 - q - r + s)^{c00-1}(r - s)^{c01-1}(q - s)^{c10-1}s^{c11-1} \times (\min\{q, r\}) - \max\{0 + q + r - 1\}).$$

As can be seen in the online materials, this can be implemented in just a couple of lines of R code.

We apply this algorithm to some synthetically generated datasets when the chosen prior distribution is based on $c_{00} = c_{01} = c_{10} = c_{11} = 2$, and the data are simulated under the conditions $Pr(X = 1) = 0.2$ and $Pr(Y = 1) = 0.2$. Note that these settings correspond to the leftmost LPD in Figure 2.1. A telescoping data sequence is generated, with "stops" at $n_x = n_y = n$, for $n = 10$, $n = 40$, $n = 160$, and $n = 640$. This choice is rather deliberate, since we are accustomed to seeing statistical procedures with $\sqrt{n}$ performance, in the sense that uncertainty is reduced by a factor of two upon a fourfold increase in sample size. The posterior distribution of p_{11} at each of our stops is portrayed in Figure 2.2. We see that $n = 10$ datapoints gets us to a posterior distribution which is noticeably sharper than the prior distribution, and just $n = 40$ datapoints appears to get us more than halfway along our journey from the prior distribution to the limiting posterior distribution. The next quadrupling of sample size, to $n = 160$, does not yield very much further concentration of the posterior, but it does get us to something nearly as concentrated as the limiting posterior. Finally, with $n = 640$ we have a posterior that is just as concentrated as the limiting posterior, but is not quite centered in the same place. Of course this occurs as the sample prevalences of t_x/n_x and t_y/n_y are slightly off from the corresponding population prevalences for X and Y. The overarching impression from Figure 2.2 though is one of diminishing returns. Even a modest amount of data gives us a posterior distribution nearly as concentrated as the limiting posterior distribution. Further data acquisition beyond this point will have very little impact on the investigator's knowledge about the target.

Of course, with any results based on simulated data, it is sensible to ask to what extent are results specific to the realized data values, rather than general, at least for the settings giving rise to the simulated datasets. Given this, in Figure 2.3 we redo Figure 2.2 for a freshly simulated data sequence. Importantly, we note the message concerning the diminishing returns of collecting more than a modest amount of data is unchanged.

Before moving on from this example, we pick up on a couple of issues. First, we consider the extent to which the posterior distribution is sensitive to the prior distribution. Referring back to Figure 2.1, we saw the shape of the LPD arising under selected parameter values, for the prior distribution corresponding to hyperparameters $(c_{00}, c_{01}, c_{10}, c_{11}) = (2, 2, 2, 2)$. It was already mentioned that a flatter prior based on $(c_{00}, c_{01}, c_{10}, c_{11}) = (1, 1, 1, 1)$ induces a uniform LPD over the identification interval, i.e., we would see much "shorter and squatter" distributions relative to those in Figure 2.1. To explore this further, in Figure 2.4 we show the LPDs arising for some further choices of hyperparameters. While of course the choice of prior has no influence on the *support* of the LPD, the influence on the *shape* can be quite pronounced. For instance, at least "by eye" the sharpening of the LPD seen upon increasing the

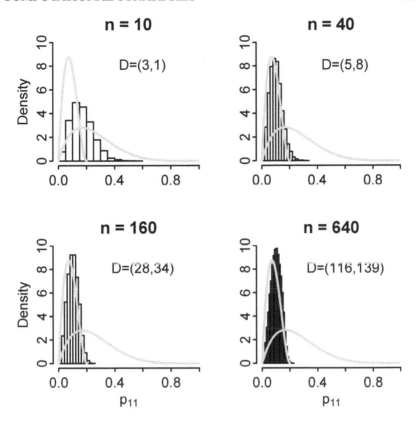

Figure 2.2 *Finite-sample posterior distribution for p_{11} in Example A, with a Dirichlet(2,2,2,2) prior on $p_{\bullet\bullet}$. In each panel the sample size $n_x = n_y = n$ is indicated, as are the simulated data values $D = (t_x, t_y)$. The true marginal prevalences are 0.2 for both X and Y. For reference, the dotted curves in each panel give the prior and limiting posterior distributions of the target.*

prior's effective sample size from 12 to 16 seems more pronounced than the corresponding sharpening of the prior marginal distribution (from Beta(3,9) to Beta(4,12)).

A final point to dwell upon is that one would often like to understand the loss incurred in having limited data rather than ideal or "full" data. To explore this, we simulate full data in the form of n observations on (X, Y). Letting t_{xy} be the number of these observations for which $(X = x, Y = y)$, we immediately have the marginal posterior distribution of p_{11} given the full data as Beta$(c_{11} + t_{11}, c_{00} + c_{01} + c_{10} + n - t_{11})$. We compare this ideal or "full" posterior distribution to the "limited" posterior arising from marginal data only. In particular, we take $t_x = t_{x0} + t_{x1}$ to be the marginal count of $X = 1$ from the

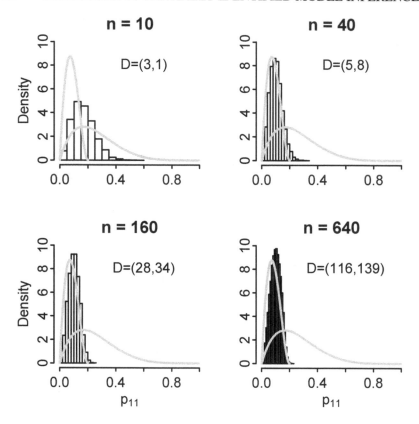

Figure 2.3 *Finite-sample posterior distribution for p_{11} in Example A, with a Dirichlet(2,2,2,2) prior on $p_{\bullet\bullet}$. The settings and layout are as per Figure 2.2, but a freshly simulated data sequence is used.*

full data, but then simulate t_y as the marginal count of $Y = 1$ from a freshly drawn sample, of size n. Fixing $n = 100$ and $(c_{00}, c_{01}, c_{10}, c_{11}) = (1,1,1,1)$, Figure 2.5 compares the "full" and "limited" posterior distributions on p_{11}, for four replications of the data-generating scheme. By eye, the reduction in information for the limited scheme is on the order of a factor of two, in terms of the width and height of the posterior density. We redo the comparison for $n = 400$ in Figure 2.6. Unsurprisingly, the contrast between the full and limited posterior distributions is even starker now. Of course this happens because the quadrupling of sample size induces a factor of two improvement in the width of the full posterior distribution, but only a very modest improvement in the limited posterior distribution. ∎

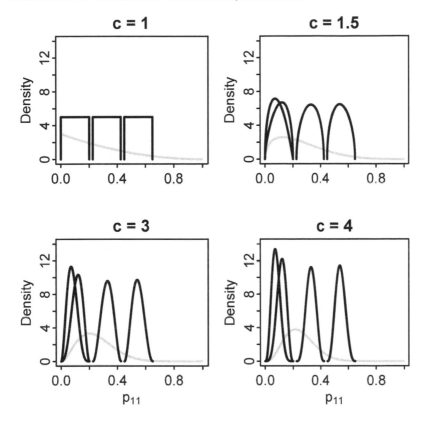

Figure 2.4 *The influence of the prior on the limiting posterior distribution in Example A. The underlying marginal prevalences are as per Figure 2.1. The prior distribution is $p_{\bullet\bullet} \sim Dirichlet(c,c,c,c)$, for selected values of c.*

2.4   Strength of Bayesian Updating, Revisited

Example A also prompts reflection upon the different ways in which knowledge of ϕ can determine the shape of the LPD over the identification region. This reflection spawns a definition.

Consider a partially identified model with a prior π and inferential target ψ such that strong indirect learning about ψ is manifested. Let $R = R(\phi)$ be the identification region for the target, i.e., R is the support of $\pi(\psi|\phi)$. We will say that **the data speak softly** if ψ and ϕ are conditionally independent given R, and that **the data speak loudly** otherwise.

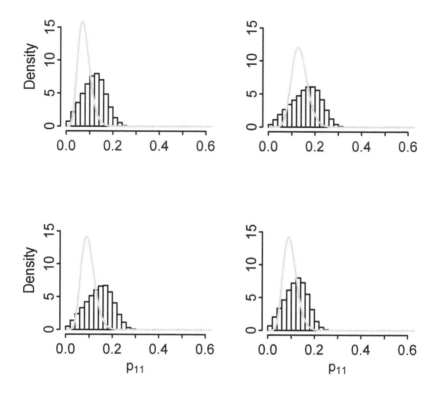

Figure 2.5 *Comparing inference from limited data and ideal data in Example A. The ideal data consist of* $n = 100$ *bivariate observations of* (X, Y). *The limited data consist of the same* $n = 100$ *observations of* X *independent from* $n = 100$ *observations of* Y. *Each panel corresponds to a replicate of the data generation, with the histogram and density curve respectively giving the limited-data and full-data posterior distributions on* $\psi = p_{11}$. *Hyperparameters are set as* $(c_{00}, c_{01}, c_{10}, c_{11}) = (1, 1, 1, 1)$.

Note the practical content of this definition. If the data speak softly, then ϕ, representing what is learned from the data, influences the LPD of ψ only through R. So two unique values of ϕ giving rise to the same identification region also give rise to the same LPD. That is, a unique LPD corresponds to a given identification region. Conversely, if the data speak loudly, then multiple values of ϕ can give rise to the same identification region but different limiting posterior distributions.

We will tend to keep an eye out for situations where the data speak loudly, as they do in Example A. They provide an interesting challenge conceptually. A non-Bayesian view suggests that the identification region itself is the tar-

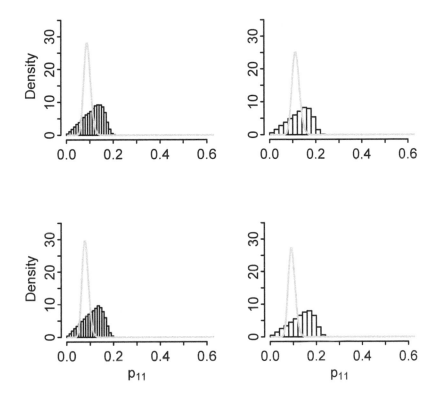

Figure 2.6 *Comparing inference from limited data and ideal data in Example A. The ideal data consist of $n = 400$ bivariate observations of (X,Y). The limited data consist of the same $n = 400$ observations of X independent from $n = 400$ observations of Y. Each panel corresponds to a replicate of the data generation, with the histogram and density curve respectively giving the limited-data and full-data posterior distributions on $\psi = p_{11}$. Hyperparameters are set as $(c_{00}, c_{01}, c_{10}, c_{11}) = (1, 1, 1, 1)$.*

get of interest, and there cannot be anything more to say once this region is determined. However, a situation where the data speak loudly is such that the data do indeed contribute more than just the determination of the identification region. This issue is explored in depth in Gustafson (2014).

The distinction between softly and loudly speaking data completes the story from Section 2.2 about the strength of Bayesian updating. In particular, we can now give a rather complete taxonomy of Bayesian inference, via the tree depicted in Figure 2.7. By starting at the top of the tree and tracing down to the appropriate leaf, we can classify a given problem in terms of the strength of Bayesian inference about the target parameter.

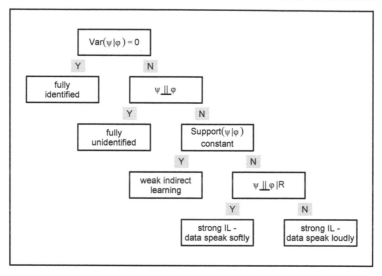

Figure 2.7 *Taxonomy of Bayesian inference. Starting at the top of the tree, one can trace down to the appropriate leaf corresponding to the strength of Bayesian updating about the target parameter ψ. The parameter φ is the identified component of a transparent parameterization, while R = R(φ) is the identification region for the target. Note that all statements concerning variance, support, and independence are with respect to the prior distribution.*

2.5   Posterior Moments

Posterior Mean as a Point Estimate

The particular structure of the limiting posterior distribution of the target parameter has implications for summaries such as the moments of this distribution. Toward determining the posterior mean of the target, let

$$
\begin{aligned}
g_\pi(\phi) &= E_\pi(\psi^\star|\phi) \\
&= \int g(\phi,\lambda)\pi(\lambda|\phi)d\lambda.
\end{aligned}
$$

Clearly then

$$
\begin{aligned}
E_\pi(\psi^\star|d_n) &= E_\pi\{E_\pi(\psi^\star|\phi^\star,d_n)|d_n\} \\
&= E_\pi\{E_\pi(\psi^\star|\phi^\star)|d_n\} \\
&= E_\pi\{g_\pi(\phi^\star)|d_n\}, \tag{2.7}
\end{aligned}
$$

from which it follows that

$$
\lim_{n\to\infty} E(\psi^\star|d_n^\star) = g_\pi\left(\phi^\dagger\right).
$$

Note that here the convergence can be interpreted as almost surely, i.e., with probability one under the distribution of data sequences $d_n^\star$ generated under the parameter values $\theta = \theta^\dagger$.

The form of (2.7) gives us some perspective. The posterior mean of the quantity of interest $g(\phi, \lambda)$ is identically the posterior mean of another quantity $g_\pi(\phi)$. Since the latter is free of λ, and since the model for the data given ϕ is a regular parametric model, at least from a point-estimation standpoint one is "in the game." Standard parametric theory dictates that the estimator will converge to $g_\pi(\phi^\dagger)$ at a $n^{1/2}$ rate. The bad news, of course, is that this limiting value is the wrong answer! The investigator wants to estimate $\psi^\dagger = g(\phi^\dagger, \lambda^\dagger)$, but ends up estimating $g_\pi(\phi^\dagger)$. Thus the price to be paid due to a lack of identification is a large-sample bias.

The large-sample bias of the posterior mean of the target depends on both the parameter values θ and the choice of prior π according to

$$
\begin{aligned}
\text{bias}(\theta; \pi) &= \lim_{n \to \infty} E_\pi(\psi^\star \mid d_n^\star) - \psi \\
&= g_\pi(\phi) - g(\phi, \lambda).
\end{aligned}
$$

The knee-jerk response to an estimation bias that does not go away as the sample size increases is that the estimator in question is worthless. We must be more circumspect, however. First, the very nature of nonidentification implies immediately that consistent estimation is impossible, since multiple values of the target are consistent with the law of the observed data. Second, there is a huge distinction between biases which are unacknowledged and those which are acknowledged. By unacknowledged bias we refer to a situation where the estimator converges to the wrong value as the sample size grows, while its accompanying measure of uncertainty goes to zero. Clearly this would be misleading: as the sample size increases, ever more confidence is imbued in a wrong answer. Fortunately, consideration of posterior variance shows us that Bayesian inference in a partially identified model involves *acknowledged* bias.

Posterior Variance as an Uncertainty Estimate

Along the lines of (2.7), the posterior variance of the target can be decomposed as follows.

$$
\begin{aligned}
\text{Var}_\pi(\psi^\star | d_n) &= E_\pi\{\text{Var}_\pi(\psi^\star | \phi^\star, d_n) | d_n\} + \text{Var}_\pi\{E_\pi(\psi^\star | \phi^\star, d_n) | d_n\} \\
&= E_\pi\{\text{Var}_\pi(\psi^\star | \phi^\star) | d_n\} + \text{Var}_\pi\{E_\pi(\psi^\star | \phi^\star) | d_n\}.
\end{aligned}
$$

Note that the second term could be reexpressed as the posterior variance of $g_\pi(\phi)$, which, according to standard theory, will fall off like n^{-1}. The first term, however, acknowledges the bias by tending to a positive value as the sample size grows. We can summarize as follows.

The bias of $E_\pi(\psi^*|d_n^*)$ as an estimator of ψ is acknowledged by a posterior variance which will not tend to zero as the sample size increases. Particularly,

$$\lim_{n\to\infty} \text{Var}_\pi(\psi^*|d_n^*) = \text{Var}_\pi(\psi^*|\phi^* = \phi^\dagger)$$

$$= \int \{g(\phi^\dagger,\lambda) - g_\pi(\phi^\dagger)\}^2 \pi(\lambda|\phi^\dagger)d\lambda.$$

Note the intuitive form here. The uncertainty remaining after observing an infinite data sample is based on the average squared difference between the target $g(\phi,\lambda)$ and the unintended estimand $g_\pi(\phi)$, with ϕ pinned down at the true value $\phi^\dagger$, as learned from the data.

Example A, Continued

Consider the simplest case of the Dirichlet$(1,1,1,1)$ prior distribution on the cell probabilities $p_{xy} = Pr(X = x, Y = y)$, so that the LPD for the target parameter $\psi = p_{11}$ is simply a uniform distribution over the identification region. Recall that the identification region for ψ is the interval running from $\max(0, q+r-1)$ to $\min(q, r)$, where $q = p_{1+} = Pr(X = 1)$ and $r = p_{+1} = Pr(Y = 1)$. The mean and variance of the LPD are thus

$$\mu(q,r) = (1/2)\{\max(0, q+r-1) + \min(q, r)\}$$

and

$$v(q,r) = (1/12)\{\min(q, r) - \max(0, q+r-1)\}^2,$$

respectively.

For finite samples, along the lines of (2.2),

$$E(\psi^*|d_n) = E\{\mu(q^*, r^*)|d_n\},$$
$$Var(\psi^*|d_n) = E\{v(q^*, r^*)|d_n\} + Var\{\mu(q^*, r^*)|d_n\}.$$

For a given dataset d_n these moments can be computed via two-dimensional numerical integration. Recall that data arrive in the form of t_x of n_x subjects having $X = 1$, and independently t_y of n_y subjects having $Y = 1$. Marginalizing $\pi(q, r, s)$ as given in (2.4) yields

$$\pi(q, r) \quad \propto \quad 0.5 - \max\{|q - 0.5|, |r - 0.5|\},$$

which can be visualized as a pyramidal density on the unit square. A convenient integration scheme arises from the proportionality of the likelihood function $q^{t_x}(1 - q)^{n_x - t_x} r^{t_y}(1 - r)^{n_y - t_y}$ with the product of two beta densities. For any function $f()$,

$$E\{f(q^\star, r^\star)|d_n\} \quad = \quad \frac{E_n^*\{f(q^\star, r^\star)\pi(q^\star, r^\star)\}}{E_n^*\{\pi(q^\star, r^\star)\}},$$

with E_n^* denoting expectation with respect to $q^\star \sim Beta(t_x + 1, n_x - t_x + 1)$ independently of $r^\star \sim Beta(t_y + 1, n_y - t_y - 1)$. Thus a quadrature scheme using say quantiles of these distributions is very easily applied.

Figure 2.8 displays the evolution of the posterior mean and posterior standard deviation as data accumulate, for five simulated data series. The two samples are taken to be equal-sized, i.e., $n_x = n_y = n$, and the posterior moments are reported for five values as n grows. The prior moments ($n = 0$) and the LPD moments ($n \to \infty$) are also given. The data are simulated under $q^\dagger = 0.425$ and $r^\dagger = 0.8$, corresponding to the identification region $p_{11} \in (0.225, 0.425)$.

As theory dictates, the posterior mean evolves toward its large-sample limit in the manner of an ordinary estimator in a parametric model. The posterior SD, however, has the tell-tale signature of partial identification. It decreases initially, but then stabilizes at a relatively small sample size. In this case there is almost no further reduction in posterior SD beyond $n = 200$. And for n smaller than this, the uncertainty is being reduced at a slower rate than seen in identified settings. Specifically, we see a quadrupling of sample size yielding a reduction in posterior SD by much *less* than a factor of two. ■

2.6 Credible Intervals

Preliminaries

While the posterior SD is an intuitive and mathematically convenient summary of the *a posteriori* uncertainty about a target parameter, in applications one more commonly sees this uncertainty reflected by a posterior credible interval. As a standard Bayesian tool, having observed data d_n, a $(1 - \alpha)$ posterior credible interval for target parameter ψ is simply an interval having probability $1 - \alpha$ under the posterior marginal distribution, $\pi(\psi|d_n)$. The nature of the Bayesian framework imbues a direct interpretation for credible intervals. For instance, if a 95% credible interval for ψ is determined to be $(2.1, 4.7)$, we can ascribe 95% probability to $2.1 < \psi < 4.7$ being a true statement. That is, while

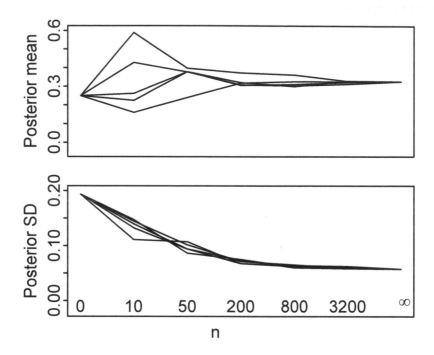

Figure 2.8 *Evolution of the posterior mean (top) and posterior standard deviation (SD) (bottom) in Example A, as data accumulate. Results are based on five data series simulated under* $(q^{\dagger}, r^{\dagger}) = (0.425, 0.8)$. *The posterior moments are computed at the five values of n indicated, as well as n = 0 (the prior) and n → ∞ (the LPD).*

the statement must be either true or false, based on the evidence contained in the data we perceive it 19 times more likely to be true than to be false. Of course this is a substantial point of departure from frequentist confidence intervals. If a frequentist confidence interval is determined to be $(2.1, 4.7)$, it is meaningless to refer to any sort of "chance" that $2.1 < \psi < 4.7$, since all the constituent quantities are treated as fixed. Instead, the interpretation for frequentist confidence intervals is couched in terms of "what if" repeated datasets, and hence 95% confidence intervals, were generated under fixed parameter values. In the long run, 95% of these intervals would contain the true value of the target.

A proviso about posterior credible intervals is that they come in more than one flavor. The two most commonly seen versions are *equal-tailed* credible intervals and *highest posterior density* (HPD) posterior credible intervals. The equal-tailed $1 - \alpha$ posterior credible interval for ψ is defined as having the $\alpha/2$ and $1 - \alpha/2$ quantiles of $\pi(\psi | d_n)$ as its endpoints. Thus we discard equal amounts of posterior probability on either side of the interval. Equal-tailed posterior credible intervals are commonly used, presumably because (i), they are intuitively straightforward, (ii), they are easy to compute from MCMC output, and (iii), they possess a nice invariance property. Particularly, if $s()$ is a monotone function, then it is simple to see that the $(1 - \alpha)$ equal-tailed interval for $s(\psi)$ can be obtained as by applying $s()$ to the endpoints of the $(1 - \alpha)$ equal-tailed interval for ψ. This allows reference to "the" equal-tailed credible interval for a target parameter, without undue concern about the chosen scale on which to conduct inference.

The HPD interval is actually properly defined as a posterior credible *set*. That is, the $(1 - \alpha)$ posterior credible set for ψ is defined as $\{\psi : \pi(\psi|d_n) > c\}$, with c chosen to ensure the set indeed has probability content $1 - \alpha$ under $\pi(\psi|d_n)$. Very often the HPD credible set does indeed transpire to be an interval. Note, particularly, that this is guaranteed if $\pi(\psi|d_n)$ is a unimodal density function.

The appealing property of the HPD criterion is as follows. Should the $(1 - \alpha)$ HPD posterior credible set indeed be an interval, then it is the shortest of all intervals possessing posterior probability $1 - \alpha$. Two immediate things to note about HPD intervals are as follows. First, if $\pi(\psi|d_n)$ is a symmetric density function, then the $(1 - \alpha)$ HPD interval will coincide with the $(1 - \alpha)$ equal-tailed credible interval. Second, HPD intervals do not possess the invariance property enjoyed by equal-tailed intervals, i.e., for a monotone function $s()$ one does not in general find that the $(1 - \alpha)$ HPD credible interval for $s(\psi)$ coincides with $s()$ applied to the endpoints of the $(1 - \alpha)$ HPD credible interval for ψ. Nevertheless, in this book we focus mostly on HPD credible intervals, since we often encounter posterior marginal distributions which are far from symmetric, and the "shortest possible" consideration becomes important in this situation.

Properties of Credible Intervals

In this chapter we already have considerable experience with the limiting posterior distribution describing what happens to posterior quantities as the data accumulate. Thus the situation for credible intervals should come as no surprise. Just as we write $E_\pi()$ to denote the expectation operator applied to prior and posterior marginal distributions, we can write $H_\pi^{(\alpha)}()$ to denote the $(1 - \alpha)$ HPD operator. For instance, the 95% HPD credible interval for target parameter ψ is expressed as $H_\pi^{(0.05)}(\psi^\star | d_n^\star = d_n)$. Here we implicitly assume that $H_\pi^{(\alpha)}()$ is being applied to univariate distributions which are sufficiently smooth, i.e., have continuous density functions. Then we immediately have the following.

As the sample size grows, the $(1 - \alpha)$ HPD set will tend to the corresponding set based on the limiting posterior distribution. That is, as $n \to \infty$,

$$H_\pi^{(\alpha)} (\psi^\star | d_n^\star) \overset{\text{a.s.}}{\to} H_\pi^{(\alpha)} \left(\psi^\star | \phi^\star = \phi^\dagger \right). \tag{2.8}$$

Reflecting on the above, we start to realize that the behavior of posterior credible intervals in partially identified settings is qualitatively very distinct from the familiar "textbook" behavior of frequentist confidence intervals in identified settings. The defining property of a $(1 - \alpha)$ frequentist confidence interval is that for any fixed parameter values, and for any sample size, the chance of the generated data yielding an interval which covers the target is $1 - \alpha$. On the other hand, looking at (2.8) we realize that for the underlying parameter values $\theta^\dagger$, $\psi^\dagger$ is either in $H_\pi^{(\alpha)}(\psi^\star | \phi^\star = \phi^\dagger)$ or not. As elaborated upon in Gustafson (2012), we have the following:

Fix the prior π, and fix $\alpha \in (0, 1)$. Let $c_{\pi,n}^{(\alpha)}(\theta)$ be the frequentist coverage of the Bayesian $(1 - \alpha)$ HPD set, i.e., the probability that a dataset $d_n^\star$, generated under parameter values θ, yields an interval covering the corresponding target $\psi = \tilde{g}(\theta)$. Then

$$\lim_{n \to \infty} c_{\pi,n}^{(\alpha)}(\theta) = I\left\{ \tilde{g}(\theta) \in H_\pi^{(\alpha)}(\psi^\star | \phi^\star = \phi) \right\}. \tag{2.9}$$

The force of this statement is that as we consider ever larger sample sizes, the chance of the interval estimate covering the target goes to either zero or one. There is no middle ground.

On casual glance, this property seems like a deficiency. A frequentist $(1 - \alpha)$ confidence interval has the nicer property that the limit of its coverage probability is $(1 - \alpha)$, simply because for any finite n the coverage probability is $(1 - \alpha)$. It must be noted, however, that even schemes to construct *approximate* frequentist confidence intervals rely upon having identified models. For instance, the usual arguments yielding confidence intervals from the large-sample theory for maximum likelihood estimators are underpinned by an identification assumption. Some recent work on interval estimation in partially identified problems from a frequentist perspective includes Imbens and Manski (2004), Vansteelandt et al. (2006), Romano and Shaikh (2008), and Stoye (2009).

In fact, (2.9) suggests we think about the parameter space $\theta \in \Theta$ as being carved up into two pieces, according to whether or not (ϕ, ψ) satisfy $\psi \in$

$H_\pi^{(\alpha)}(\psi^\star|\phi^\star = \phi)$. Thus we have the "good" set of parameter values, under which the frequentist coverage of the credible interval tends to 100% as the sample size grows. The "bad" complement of this set is the values under which the frequentist coverage tends to zero.

Now, as stressed in Chapter 1, for any Bayesian model (identified or not), and any sample size (large or not), posterior credible intervals have a particular calibration property. Say $I(d_n)$ is a $(1 - \alpha)$ posterior credible interval obtained upon observing data $d_n^\star = d_n$. We can ask what is the *average* of the frequentist coverage of this procedure, where the average is with respect to the prior distribution over the parameter space. Notationally, this average is

$$
\begin{aligned}
E_\pi Pr_\pi\{\psi^\star \in I(d_n^\star)|\theta^\star\} &= Pr_\pi\{\psi^\star \in I(d_n^\star)\} \\
&= E_\pi Pr_\pi\{\psi^\star \in I(d_n^\star)|d_n^\star\} \\
&= E_\pi(1 - \alpha) \\
&= (1 - \alpha).
\end{aligned} \tag{2.10}
$$

That is, *any* Bayesian posterior credible interval procedure has a frequentist coverage which must *exactly* average out to the nominal (i.e., stated, or claimed) level across the parameter space, where this averaging is weighed according to the prior distribution over the parameter space.

Aside: Fundamental Calibration Property of Bayesian Credible Intervals

It is the author's contention that (2.10) is quite a fundamental operating characteristic of Bayesian procedures. It is hard to trace its roots in the literature though, and sadly it gets virtually no attention in most introductory books on Bayesian methods. Against that, though, it does crop up in curious circumstances. For instance, Cook et al. (2006) use it to underpin a method of software validation. That is, they propose checking computer code to calculate posterior quantities, by making sure that simulation results are consistent with (2.10).★

Getting back to (2.9) and the notion of the "good-bad" partition of the parameter space, (2.10) tells us something. Since it holds exactly, at any sample size, it must also hold in the large-sample limit. The 100% limiting frequentist coverage for θ values in the good set must then average with the 0% for the complementary bad set in a way that arrives at $(1 - \alpha) \times 100\%$ aggregate coverage. So the good set *must* have prior probability $(1 - \alpha)$ and its complement must have prior probability α. This gives a sense in which the subset of the parameter space for which the interval estimator performs badly is small. Gustafson (2012) takes a deeper look at this situation, with particular focus on where in the parameter space the "bad" set lies.

Example A, Continued

To visualize some posterior credible intervals, we return to our ecological inference example. We use the prior specification $p_{xy} \sim$ Dirichlet$(2,2,2,2)$, and determine the resulting HPD intervals for $\psi = p_{11}$ (at the 50%, 80% and 95% levels) for three different telescoping data sequences. Each sequence starts with $n = n_x = n_y = 25$, and involves five successive quadruplings to $n = 6400$. The first of these data streams is generated under marginal X and Y prevalences of $(p_{1+}, p_{+1}) = (0.8, 0.15)$, while the second and third use $(0.5, 0.5)$, and $(0.95, 0.15)$, respectively.

The HPD intervals appear in Figure 2.9. The corresponding *prior* highest-density intervals associated with the marginal prior $p_{11} \sim$ beta$(2,6)$ are also displayed, as are the intervals associated with the LPD. The example serves to illustrate that depending on the underlying parameter values, the extent to which knowledge is gained as data accumulate could be minimal (see the middle panel), substantial (see the lower panel), or somewhere in between (see the upper panel). It also serves to remind us that the first datapoints may be quite informative, but then are followed with diminishing returns. That is, it can be a relatively small sample size at which the credible interval becomes almost as narrow as its large-sample limit.■

Aside: Visualizing a Distribution Through Credible Intervals

The display of HPD intervals at multiple levels in Figure 2.9 is set up in a rather deliberate fashion. The three intervals are depicted as adjacent rectangles of varying widths, with these widths chosen such that taken together the rectangles can be viewed as a rough depiction of the density, turned sideways. This is easily achieved, as follows. Say in general there are k credible intervals based on $\alpha_1 < \alpha_2 < \ldots < \alpha_k$, with their corresponding lengths necessarily ordered as $l_1 > l_2 > \ldots l_k$. Letting $w_1, \ldots, w_k$ denote the rectangle widths, then, turned sideways, the total area "under the curve" for the j-th interval will be $(w_1 + \ldots + w_j)l_j + w_{j+1}l_{j+1} + \ldots w_k l_k$. Thus by taking

$$
\begin{pmatrix} w_1 \\ \ldots \\ w_k \end{pmatrix} \propto \begin{pmatrix} l_1 & l_2 & l_3 & \ldots & l_{k-1} & l_k \\ l_2 & l_2 & l_3 & \ldots & l_{k-1} & l_k \\ l_3 & l_3 & l_3 & \ldots & l_{k-1} & l_k \\ & & & \ldots & & \\ l_{k-1} & l_{k-1} & l_{k-1} & \ldots & l_{k-1} & l_k \\ l_k & l_k & l_k & \ldots & l_k & l_k \end{pmatrix}^{-1} \begin{pmatrix} 1 - \alpha_1 \\ \ldots \\ 1 - \alpha_k \end{pmatrix},
$$

we achieve the desired property. That is, the areas corresponding to the intervals are in proportion to the probability content of the intervals. As per Figure 2.9, we will make future use of this graphical device to convey a posterior marginal distribution via credible intervals, along with an indication of the

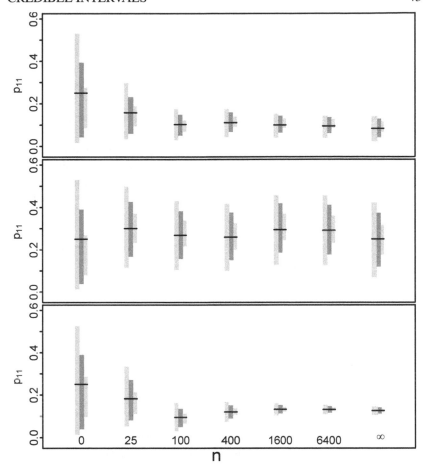

Figure 2.9 *Evolution of HPD credible intervals for p_{11} in Example A. The three data streams are generated under marginal prevalences of* $(0.8, 0.15)$ *(top panel),* $(0.5, 0.5)$ *(middle panel), and* $(0.95, 0.15)$ *(lower panel). The results include the highest prior density interval* $(n = 0)$, *and the LPD intervals* $(n = \infty)$. *In every instance, 50%, 80%, and 95% intervals are displayed, and the posterior mean is also marked.*

posterior mean. When $k = 3$ and $(\alpha_1, \alpha_2, \alpha_3) = (0.05, 0.2, 0.5)$, we will refer to such a display as a *tri-interval* plot. ★

Example A, Continued

We also take a look at the frequentist coverage of credible intervals in this example. Consider three different θ settings: (i) $p_{xy} = (0.18, 0.67, 0.02, 0.13)$, (ii)

$p_{xy} = (0.15, 0.7, 0.05, 0.1)$, and (iii) $p_{xy} = (0.105, 0.745, 0.095, 0.055)$. Note that all three induce the same marginal prevalences of $p_{1+} = 0.8$ for X and $p_{+1} = 0.15$ for Y. In fact, this is the intermediate case in Figure 2.9, in terms of how much knowledge accumulates as the sample size grows. For each setting, and for a variety of sample sizes, we compute the frequentist coverage of the 80% HPD interval for p_{11}. This is simply done empirically, i.e., by repeatedly simulating a dataset, computing the HPD interval, and checking whether it contains the target. (A shortcut ensues, as the same set of simulated datasets speak to all three parameter settings, since they all have the same marginal prevalences.) The results appear in Figure 2.10. We see empirical confirmation of the behavior described above theoretically. For parameter settings (i) and (ii), the frequentist coverage tends to 100% as the sample size grows, while for setting (iii) it tends to 0%.■

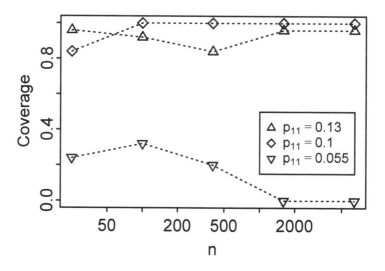

Figure 2.10 *Frequentist coverage of 80% credible intervals for selected sample sizes n, in Example A. The underlying parameter values are $p_{1+} = 0.80$, $p_{+1} = 0.15$, and (i) $p_{11} = 0.055$, (ii) $p_{11} = 0.10$, and (iii) $p_{11} = 0.13$. Note the use of a logarithmic axis for n. Each reported coverage probability is based on 400 simulated datasets, hence all Monte Carlo standard errors are less than 0.025*

2.7   Evaluating the Worth of Inference

Preliminaries

Toward further understanding the "information flow" in partially identified models, we now consider what happens to the mean-squared error (MSE) of an estimator as the data accumulate. Using the posterior mean of the target ψ as our estimator, with data d_n we incur an estimation error of $E(\psi^\star|d_n) - \psi^\dagger$. In terms of a transparent parameterization then, the mean-squared error arising over repeated instantiations of the data, with the parameters fixed, can be written as

$$MSE_{n,\pi}(\phi^\dagger, \lambda^\dagger) \quad = \quad E_\pi\left[\left\{E(\psi^\star|d_n^\star) - g(\phi^\dagger, \lambda^\dagger)\right\}^2 \Big| \phi^\star = \phi^\dagger, \lambda^\star = \lambda^\dagger\right].$$

By the arguments given earlier in this chapter, as n increases this tends to

$$MSE_{\infty,\pi}(\phi^\dagger, \lambda^\dagger) \quad = \quad \left\{g_\pi(\phi^\dagger) - g(\phi^\dagger, \lambda^\dagger)\right\}^2. \tag{2.11}$$

Of course, (2.11) reflects estimator bias only, as the estimator variance falls away with sample size.

Now, think of (2.11) as a function across the parameter space, i.e., $MSE_{\infty,\pi}(\phi, \lambda)$ describes estimator performance as the underlying values of (ϕ, λ) vary. In our experience, many partially identified situations involve the MSE varying strongly across the parameter space, to an extent which would be uncommon in identified model settings. A natural desire is to somehow average the performance across the parameter space. Harkening back to Section 1.3, a rather general way to do this would be to consider *two* distributions across the parameter space. Let the *investigator's prior distribution* π_I be the prior distribution used to form posterior inferences, so that $MSE_{\infty,\pi_I}()$ describes the limiting estimator performance across different values of the underlying parameters. And say we are interested in weighting our summary of performance using the distribution π_N across the parameter space. We can term π_N as "Nature's parameter-generating distribution," or simply "Nature's prior," with the notion that we are measuring aggregate performance across a sequence of *different* studies with different true values of the parameters. That is, for each study $\theta^\star$ is drawn afresh from π_N. Then $E_{\pi_N}\{MSE_{\infty,\pi_I}(\phi^\star, \lambda^\star)\}$ would summarize the aggregate performance.

An important special case is when the two distributions over the parameter space agree, i.e., $\pi_N = \pi_I$, with the common distribution simply denoted as π. This puts us squarely in the realm of the decision-theoretic view of statistical inference, with the aggregate estimator performance referred to as the *Bayes risk* (BR). For a finite sample size n we write

$$BR_{n,\pi} \quad = \quad E_\pi\{MSE_{n,\pi}(\phi^\star, \lambda^\star)\}, \tag{2.12}$$

and analogously for the large-sample limit:

$$BR_{\infty,\pi} \quad = \quad E_\pi\{MSE_{\infty,\pi}(\phi^\star, \lambda^\star)\}. \tag{2.13}$$

Aside: A Blurb on Decision Theory

In fact, (2.12) is the Bayes risk for a specific choice of *loss function*—the squared error loss, and a specific estimator—the posterior mean. More generally, one can write $L\{\tilde{g}(\theta), \delta(d_n)\}$ as the loss incurred when the target, $\tilde{g}(\theta)$, is estimated by some function of the data, $\delta(d_n)$. Then the Bayes risk of this particular estimator is $E_\pi L\{\tilde{g}(\theta^\star), \delta(d_n^\star)\}$. The decision-theoretic optimality of Bayesian procedures is manifested by the fact that amongst all possible estimators, the one with smallest Bayes risk is given by

$$\delta(d_n) \;=\; \text{argmin}_a E_\pi \left[L\{\tilde{g}(\theta^\star), a\} | d_n^\star = d_n \right].$$

Thus, for a given value of the data, the best guess at the target is that which makes the posterior expected loss smallest. In the case of squared-error loss this simply devolves to the best guess being the posterior mean of the target.

The decision-theoretic view adds richness to the case for using Bayesian methods. One can simply view the investigator as providing a "weighting function," describing how much weight parameter values should get relative to one another when aggregating estimator performance across the parameter space. Then we find that the optimal strategy is to use this weighting function as a prior density and carry out *a posteriori* inference. This is in contrast with axiomatic developments of subjective probability, where the prior distribution is viewed as coherently capturing beliefs in terms of which gambles concerning the true parameter values seem favorable to the investigator. For more on the decision-theoretic underpinnings of the Bayesian approach, see Berger (1985) and Bernardo and Smith (1994). ★

Coming back to (2.13), we immediately have

$$BR_{\infty,\pi} \;=\; E_\pi \left[\{ g_\pi(\phi^\star) - g(\phi^\star, \lambda^\star) \}^2 \right]. \tag{2.14}$$

Intuitively this makes perfect sense. In the large-sample limit, with random-sampling variation no longer at issue, the aggregate performance is simply the across-parameter average of the squared difference between the estimand forced upon us due to the lack of identification and the estimand of real interest.

At the study-planning stage, with a model and prior formulated but no data yet collected, one strategy would be to evaluate (2.14) as a measure of how well one anticipates estimating the target from an infinite amount of data. If (2.14) turns out to be impractically large, then it may be appropriate to recommend *against* continuing to the stage of actual data collection, i.e., no amount of data could provide a usefully narrow answer. On the other hand, if the size of (2.14) is tolerable, then the next question is: how large a value of (2.12) is acceptable. Necessarily (2.12) is larger than (2.14), but the difference between them can be made as small as desired upon the choice of a sufficiently large sample size. Such study design questions will be taken up later in this book.

Logarithmic Scoring

We have seen a decision-theoretic sense in which the typical closeness of the posterior mean $E(\psi^\star | d_n)$ to the estimand $\psi^\dagger$ summarizes the worth of point estimation. In an analogous fashion, the typical *height* of the posterior marginal density $\pi(\psi|d_n)$, evaluated at the estimand $\psi^\dagger$ speaks to the worth of a distributional estimator. Again referring to decision theory, the posterior marginal density of the target minimizes the Bayes risk under a logarithmic scoring loss, just as the posterior mean of the target minimizes the Bayes risk under squared-error loss. That is, amongst all families of densities for ψ indexed by d_n, written generically as $f(\psi; d_n)$, we prefer $E_\pi\{\log f(\psi^\star; d_n^\star)\}$ to be as large as possible. It is straightforward to see that the Bayesian posterior distribution of ψ is indeed optimal. If the choice $f(\psi; d_n) = \pi(\psi|d_n)$ were beaten by a different choice $f^*(\psi; d_n)$, then immediately

$$\int \int \log \frac{\pi(\psi|d_n)}{f^*(\psi; d_n)} d\Pi(\psi|d_n) \, d\Pi(d_n) \quad < \quad 0. \qquad (2.15)$$

Here, however, the inner integral is the Kullback-Leibler divergence between two density functions, which, by definition, is non-negative. Hence (2.15) cannot arise.

Proceeding, we can write the minimized Bayes risk as

$$BR_{n,\pi} \quad = \quad E_\pi\{\log \pi(\psi^\star|d_n^\star)\},$$

and then pass to the large-sample limit as

$$BR_{\infty,\pi} \quad = \quad E_\pi\{\log \pi(\psi^\star|\phi^\star)\}. \qquad (2.16)$$

So the information lost when something other than the LPD is used to infer the target from an infinite dataset is quantified as follows. Take

$$\Delta \quad = \quad 1 - \exp\left[E_\pi\{\log f(\psi^\star; \phi^\star) - \log \pi(\psi^\star|\phi^\star)\}\right]. \qquad (2.17)$$

Then the typical height of the limiting "density estimate" $f(\psi; \phi)$ evaluated at the target is $100 \times \Delta$ percent lower than the typical height of the LPD evaluated at the target.

As emphasized in Gustafson (2014), (2.17) opens a route to saying how useful the "shape" of the limiting posterior distribution is, beyond simply finding the identification region. In particular, one can compare the LPD to other distributions over the identification region. Such comparisons seem particularly relevant in order to contrast with non-Bayesian approaches to partial identification. Without Bayes, the feeling is that all the data can do is locate the identification region, without conveying any sense that some values in the region are more plausible than others.

One possible competitor to the LPD would be the marginal prior density of ψ truncated to the identification region $R(\phi)$, formally expressed as

$$f(\psi; \phi) \quad = \quad \frac{\pi(\psi)I\{\psi \in R(\phi)\}}{\int_{R(\phi)} \pi(\tilde\psi) d\tilde\psi}.$$

This combines the information arriving via ϕ and the *a priori* weighting of target values ψ in a naïve way. Another simple alternative is a uniform distribution over the identification region.

We have already touched upon the subtlety that in the face of strong indirect learning, the data may speak "softly" or "loudly" about the target. If the data speak only softly then the shape of the LPD may vary *across*, but not *within*, identification regions. To be more precise, consider the situation where $R(\phi)$ is an interval, for all ϕ. For either softly or loudly speaking data, if $R(\phi_1) \neq R(\phi_2)$, then $\pi(\psi|\phi_2)$ may not be merely a simple transform (e.g., location-scale) of $\pi(\psi|\phi_1)$. So the effect of the data on the LPD can be more nuanced than simply "rescaling" the answer to fit on the appropriate identification region. Thus we say the shape of the LPD can vary across identification regions. On the other hand, if the data only speak softly, then immediately we have that $R(\phi_1) = R(\phi_2)$ implies $\pi(\psi|\phi_1) = \pi(\psi|\phi_2)$, so that within-region variation in the LPD is ruled out.

The following definition helps to untangle the shape and the support of the LPD.

Let the prior distribution of the target given the true identification region, i.e., the distribution of $\{\psi^\star | R(\phi^\star) = R(\phi^\dagger)\}$ under π, be referred to as the **coarsened limiting posterior distribution** (CLPD). Here "coarsened" refers to the fact that in general conditioning on R only, rather than on ϕ, corresponds to using only *some* of the information available from an infinite data stream. The definition is uninteresting when the data speak softly, since the CLPD and the LPD agree in this setting. Generally they will not agree, however, when the data speak loudly.

In problems where the data speak loudly, comparing the LPD and the CLPD is a way of quantifying the utility of the "within identification region" variation in the LPD. The CLPD gets as close to the LPD as possible while being constrained to not vary if R were fixed. Thus comparing the LPD and CLPD using (2.17) speaks to the utility of the data being able to discriminate somewhat between sets of parameter values that give rise to the same identification region.

Example A, Continued

Returning to our ecologic inference example, and again using the Dirichlet(2,2,2,2) prior on the cell probabilities p_{xy}, we consider the information loss (2.17) relative to the limiting posterior $\pi(\psi|\phi^\dagger)$ for (i) the coarsened limiting posterior $\pi(\psi|R^\dagger)$, (ii) the marginal prior for ψ truncated to the identification interval, (iii) the uniform distribution over the identification interval, and (iv) the marginal prior for ψ, i.e., untruncated.

The CLPD in this example can be understood as follows. An infinite dataset determines the identification region according to the map from $\phi = (q, r)$ to $R = (\max\{0, q + r - 1\}, \min\{q, r\})$. If the left endpoint of the identification interval is positive, then the two endpoints determine both $\min\{q, r\}$ and $\max\{q, r\}$, which, according to (2.5), suffices to uniquely determine $\pi(\psi | \phi)$, at least for hyperparameter settings with $c_{01} = c_{10}$. Thus, if the left endpoint of the identification region is positive, the CLPD and LPD agree.

Conversely, learning that the identification region is $(0, b)$ (with $b < 0.5$ necessarily), corresponds to knowledge that $\min\{q, r\} = b$ and $\max\{q, r\} \in (b, 1 - b)$. In this case, integrating (2.5) gives

$$\pi(\psi | \min\{q, r\} - b, \max\{q, r\} < 1 - b) \quad \propto$$
$$\left[\tfrac{1-b}{2}\{(1 - b - \psi)^2 - (b - \psi)^2\} + \tfrac{1}{3}\{(b - \psi)^3 - (1 - b - \psi)^3\} \right] \times$$
$$\psi(b - \psi)I\{0 < \psi < b\}.$$

Numerical evaluation of (2.17) simply proceeds by using a large number of realizations of $\theta^\star \sim \pi$, to approximate the expectation involved with a Monte Carlo average. Via the Delta method, a Monte Carlo standard error (MCSE) is easily obtained. Results appear in Table 2.1. The utility of the LPD beyond simply determining the identification region (IR) is evident: there is about a 12% information loss relative to the LPD if one instead simply truncates the prior on ψ to the identification region, and about a 15% loss if one imposes a uniform distribution on the region. Given the direct interpretation of the information loss in terms of reduction in typical density height at the target, these are substantial losses. Thus, if the analyst is willing to commit to a choice of π at least for purposes of evaluating performance via the Bayes risk, then it is wise to form the posterior distribution of the target with respect to this π. Note also that in comparing the marginal prior of ψ to the LPD we see around a 50% information loss. This provides a general intuition about the utility of data in the problem at hand: an infinite dataset typically doubles the height of the posterior density at the true value of the target, compared to the prior density.

Table 2.1 also indicates only a negligible loss of 0.5% upon using the CLPD rather than the LPD. Though note that the MCSE indicates the loss is computed precisely, effectively ruling out the possibility of the CLPD outperforming the LPD, as is consistent with the theory. For the present problem, then, the ability of the data to be useful via "within region" variation in the shape of the LPD is a point of theoretical curiosity, not one of practical gain. ∎

Method	Info. Loss (Δ)	(MCSE)
Coarsened limiting posterior	0.53%	(0.03%)
Prior truncated to IR	12.4%	(0.1%)
Uniform dist. on IR	15.3%	(0.1%)
Marginal prior	54.1%	(0.1%)

Table 2.1 *Information loss relative to the LPD in Example A. In each case, Δ is computed via 100,000 simulated draws from the prior distribution, and the corresponding Monte Carlo standard error (MCSE) is also reported.*

Chapter 3

Partial Identification versus Model Misspecification: Is Honesty Best?

3.1 The Siren Call of Identification

In the statistical and scientific literature as a whole, there is a huge predilection for working with identified models, given their intuitive and appealing properties. As more data are collected, we become more and more certain about the values of target quantities. Moreover, we have clear mathematical understanding about this march to certainty: the extent of our uncertainty scales inversely with the square root of the sample size. No wonder then, investigators might not always want to fully ponder whether the assumptions behind an identified model are appropriate for the subject-area problem at hand. In fact, it is common to encounter scientific articles in which all quantitative analysis is carried out using an identified model, with qualitative concern about the model assumptions raised only in passing, perhaps in the discussion section of the paper. Arguably this is too late, since the results from the identified model analysis have already been imbued as the main findings of the work.

To abstract the situation in a form amenable to mathematical analysis, say that full consideration of the uncertainties at play commits an investigator to a model $\pi(d_n|\theta)$ and a prior $\pi(\theta)$, and this yields only partial identification for the inferential target $\psi = \tilde{g}(\theta)$. However, the allure of identification may tempt the investigator to add further assumptions, perhaps overly optimistic in nature, that result in model identification. Without loss of generality, say that the parameter vector can in fact be partitioned as $\theta = (\theta_a, \theta_b)$, such that the hopeful assumptions are expressed as $\theta_b = 0$, and the resulting model, with unknown parameters θ_a only, is fully identified. As motivating examples, $\theta_b = 0$ could correspond to assuming that a variable is not susceptible to measurement error, or it could correspond to taking the values describing the extent of measurement error as known. In another context of hoping to infer causation from observational data, $\theta_b = 0$ might correspond to an assumption that there are not any unmeasured confounders. In the context of a particular variable prone to missingness, it might correspond to an assumption of "missing at random," i.e., the chance of missingness for any subject can only depend on the values of other variables for the subject, not the variable in question.

If the hopeful assumptions turn out to be correct, then the investigators are of course in good stead: they are basing inference on a model which is both correct and identified. Thus the march to certainty is also a march to truth. The posterior distribution on the target will narrow at the "root-n" rate and concentrate at the correct value. On the other hand, if the hopeful assumptions are false then the root-n march to certainty will still take place, but the value at which the posterior concentrates may be wrong. As always, if the specified model is incorrect, then resulting point estimators may be inconsistent, meaning there is an estimation bias which does not diminish as the sample size increases. In terms of extent, one can examine the magnitude of the asymptotic bias as a function of the distance of θ_b from zero. It may be that the bias is inconsequential if the optimistic assumption is close to correct. To determine whether this is so, one wants to examine the behavior of the bias in a neighborhood around $\theta_b = 0$. Generically, we refer to inference based on the hopeful assumptions as involving an *identified but possibly misspecified model* (IPMM).

On the other hand, we already know from Chapter 2 that an investigator using the partially identified model will also pay a price in terms of biased point estimation, whether or not $\theta_b = 0$ actually holds. That is, the large-sample limit of the posterior mean will generally differ from the correct value of the target. We temporarily set aside the very important distinction that any bias of a posterior mean in an IPMM analysis is unacknowledged, as the corresponding posterior variance still vanishes with sample size. Conversely, the bias of the posterior mean from the PIM analysis is acknowledged, by way of a posterior variance with a positive limit as the sample size goes to infinity. For now we focus only on bias of the posterior mean. We shall return to the issue of posterior variance later.

3.2   Comparing Bias

Concentrating just on bias alone, we can draw direct comparisons. The investigator choosing the IPMM route will incur a bias

$$b_{IPMM}(\theta) = \tilde{g}(\theta_a^*(\theta),0) - \tilde{g}(\theta_a,\theta_b), \qquad (3.1)$$

where $\theta_a^*(\theta)$ is the limiting value when estimating θ_a under the assumption that $\theta_b = 0$, when in fact the true parameter values are θ. This bias is directly comparable to the PIM bias discussed in Chapter 2. The PIM bias is most easily expressed with respect to a transparent reparameterization (ϕ,λ) under which the target is $\psi = g(\phi,\lambda)$. The limiting bias of the posterior mean is simply

$$b_{PIM}(\phi,\lambda) = g_\pi(\phi) - g(\phi,\lambda). \qquad (3.2)$$

Since (3.1) goes to zero as $\theta_b \to 0$ whereas generally (3.2) does not, the important question is how big a deviation of θ_b from zero is needed to make

(3.1) larger in magnitude than (3.2). If this arises when the deviation is small, then use of the partially identified model is supported.

Comparisons between (3.1) and (3.2) in a number of contexts have been reported in the literature, with some of these surveyed later in this chapter. First though, we work through a particular comparison in detail.

Example B: Estimating Prevalence in the Face of Missing Data

Let Y be a binary variable, with interest in estimating its population mean, or prevalence, $E(Y) = Pr(Y = 1)$, based on a random sample from the population. However, Y is subject to missingness. This could arise, for instance, by some sampled subjects refusing to participate in the study. Nonetheless, a binary co-variate X can be observed for all sampled subjects. As an example, X might be a demographic variable available directly via the sampling frame, whether or not a sampled individual consents to study participation. Let the binary indicator R indicate availability of Y, i.e., $R = 1$ if Y is measured and $R = 0$ if Y is missing. Then one way to conceptualize the data collection process is as independent and identically distributed observations of (X, R, RY). Another view is that the marginal distribution of (X, R) and the conditional distribution of $(Y|X, R = 1)$ are the entities learned via collection of data.

Let $p_{xy} = Pr(X = x, Y = y)$, for $x = 0, 1$, $y = 0, 1$. We assume the missingness process obeys

$$\text{logit } Pr(R = 1|X, Y) \quad = \quad \alpha_0 + \alpha_x(X - 1/2) + \alpha_y(Y - 1/2). \quad (3.3)$$

In doing so we are of course assuming structure. A more general form would include an interaction between X and Y, in which no restrictions would be supposed about the joint distribution of (X, Y, R). Note also that the centering of X and Y in (3.3) is used to make α_0 more generally interpretable as a parameter governing the proclivity for Y to be observed.

Within the taxonomy of missing data (see, for instance, Little and Rubin (2002)), Y is *missing completely at random* if $(\alpha_x, \alpha_y) = (0, 0)$, i.e., the propensity to participate in the study is not associated with either X or Y. If $\alpha_x \neq 0$ but $\alpha_y = 0$, then Y is *missing at random*, a classification permitting association between the missingness indicator and variables not prone to missingness. The most thorny situation is when $\alpha_y \neq 0$. This is *nonignorable missingness*, whereby the propensity for Y to be missing is influenced by the value of Y itself.

Before considering the full generality of a nonignorable missingness model, we present empirical examples of simpler analyses. Consider the synthetic data presented in Table 3.1. These were simulated under the parameter values $p_{00} = 0.585$, $p_{01} = 0.175$, $p_{10} = 0.065$, $p_{11} = 0.175$, along with $\alpha_0 = \text{logit } 0.25$, $\alpha_x = \log 2$, $\alpha_y = \log 1.4$. A number of things should be noted

R	X	$Y = 0$	$Y = 1$	Total
0	0			1851
0	1			490
1	0	297	120	417
1	1	57	185	242
Total				3000

Table 3.1 *Synthetic dataset of n = 3000 observations for Example B. The underlying parameter values are described in the text.*

about these settings. First, the choice of p gives rise to a very strong association between X and Y, with an odds ratios of $p_{00}p_{11}p_{01}^{-1}p_{10}^{-1} = 9$. Consequently there is potential for X to be predictive of Y for subjects with missing Y. Second, the value of the target parameter is $\psi = Pr(Y = 1) = p_{01} + p_{11} = 0.35$. Third, the choice of α_0 results in Y being missing for a large majority of study subjects. And, finally, the values of α_x and α_y respectively, reflect very strong and moderately strong influences of X and Y on the missingness indicator.

For the simpler analyses that follow, we do not actually need the full generality of the (p, α) parameterization. We represent the data in terms of n_{xyr} being the count of observations of the form $(X = x, Y = y, R = r)$. Further, a "+" notation indicates summation, e.g., $n_{x+r} = n_{x0r} + n_{x1r}$, and so on. About the simplest possible analysis one can imagine is a *complete-case* analysis, which completely discards the records for all subjects with missing Y and analyzes the data $(n_{001}, n_{011}, n_{101}, n_{111})$ as if they arose as a random sample from the (X, Y) distribution. This is well justified only under the MCAR assumption, which indeed postulates that the distributions of $(X, Y | R = 1)$ and (X, Y) are identical. With only the marginal distribution of Y being of interest, a Bayesian implementation of the complete-case analysis is easily described in terms of conjugate Bayesian updating for a binomial proportion. If $\psi^* \sim Beta(a, b)$ *a priori*, then $\psi^* \sim Beta(a + n_{+11}, b + n_{+01})$ *a posteriori*. In the present example, starting with a uniform prior on the target ($a = b = 1$) gives $\psi^* \sim Beta(306, 355)$ *a posteriori*. The commensurate posterior mean and 95% HPD interval appear as the leftmost entry in Figure 3.1.

We can similarly apply a simple conjugate treatment for a MAR analysis. Let $q_{xr} = Pr(X = x, R = r)$, so that a prior of the form $q_{xr}^* \sim Dirichlet(c_{xr})$ gives rise to the posterior $q_{xr}^* \sim Dirichlet(c_{xr} + n_{x+r})$. Also, define $\mu_x = Pr(Y = 1 | X = x, R = 1)$ for $x = 0, 1$, so that the prior $\mu_x^* \sim Beta(a_x, b_x)$ induces the posterior $\mu_x^* \sim Beta(a_x + n_{x11}, b_x + n_{x01})$, with q, μ_0, and μ_1 mutually independent *a posteriori*. Thus *iid* Monte Carlo sampling from the posterior distribution for (q, μ_0, μ_1) is readily implemented. A consequence of the MAR assumption is that $\mu_x = Pr(Y = 1 | X = x)$. Hence the target parameter $\psi = Pr(Y = 1)$ can be

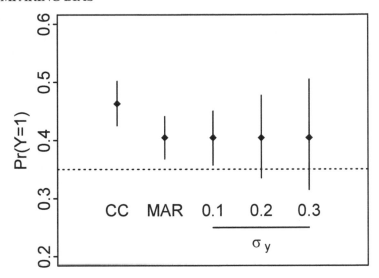

Figure 3.1 *Point and interval estimates for the prevalence of Y in Example B. The synthetic data in Table 3.1 are used. From left to right we have posterior means and 95% HPD intervals for the complete-case (CC) analysis, the MAR analysis, and three versions of the nonignorable missingness analysis with the indicated values of σ_y. The dotted line indicates the true value of the target.*

expressed as

$$\begin{aligned} \psi &= Pr(Y=1|X=0)Pr(X=0)+Pr(Y=1|X=1)Pr(X=1) \\ &= \mu_0 q_{0+}+\mu_1 q_{1+}. \end{aligned}$$

Thus a Monte Carlo sample from the posterior of (q,μ_0,μ_1) induces a Monte Carlo sample from the posterior of ψ. For the Table 3.1 data, the posterior mean and 95% HPD interval for this analysis appear in Figure 3.1 (second entry from the left). Note that the credible interval only modestly overlaps with that arising from the complete-case analysis. This underscores that the two analyses rely on different assumptions, i.e., the complete-case analysis assumes that R and Y are independent, while the MAR analysis assumes that R and Y are conditionally independent given X. Of course these data were generated in a situation where *both* these assumptions are violated, and this explains how both analyses can yield credible intervals failing to contain $\psi^\dagger = 0.35$, the true Y prevalence.

Data having missing values are often analyzed under the MAR assumption, even when the justification for the assumption is dubious. The siren call of identification is the likely culprit in this regard. For instance, returning to the (p,α) parameterization of the present problem, if α_y is assumed to be zero, then five free parameters remain: three free components of p, plus (α_0,α_x). Consistent estimation of all five is plausible, since the (X,R) marginal distribution is characterized by three probabilities and the $(Y|X, R = 1)$ conditional distribution is characterized by two probabilities. Indeed, as is implicit in the MAR analysis above, the map from the five initial parameters to these five probabilities is invertible, so that identification holds.

On the other hand, the nonignorable model, with all components of α unknown, cannot be identified. The data can only determine five quantities but there are six free parameters. Consider, then, the plight of the investigator who thinks that the MAR assumption might be close to correct, but is not able to justify its exact truth. The investigator can make the MAR assumption anyway, thereby working with a model which is identified, but perhaps incorrectly specified. This is the IPMM route. Or, the investigator can proceed with the nonignorable model, perhaps choosing a prior distribution for α_y which puts most of its mass close to zero, reflecting a supposition that a departure from MAR is unlikely to be a large departure. This is the PIM route.

To set up a transparent parameterization for this problem, it is convenient to take the initial or "scientific" parameterization to be

$$
\begin{aligned}
\theta &= (p, \mu) \\
&= (p_{01}, p_{10}, p_{11}, \mu_{01}, \mu_{10}, \mu_{11}),
\end{aligned}
$$

where, as before, $p_{xy} = Pr(X = x, Y = y)$. The elements of μ are taken as $\mu_{xy} = Pr(R = 1|X = x, Y = y)$. Of course this parameterization implicitly gives $p_{00} = 1 - p_{01} - p_{10} - p_{11}$. Similarly, the structure of (3.3) implicitly gives

$$
\mu_{00} = \text{expit} \left(\text{logit} \, \mu_{01} + \text{logit} \, \mu_{10} - \text{logit} \, \mu_{11} \right).
$$

A transparent parameterization for this problem is given as (ϕ, λ), with $\phi = (q_{01}, q_{10}, q_{11}, \gamma_{01}, \gamma_{11})$ and $\lambda = \gamma_{10}$, where

$$
\begin{aligned}
q_{xr} &= Pr(X = x, R = r) \\
&= p_{x0} \mu_{x0}^r (1 - \mu_{x0})^{1-r} + p_{x1} \mu_{x1}^r (1 - \mu_{x1})^{1-r},
\end{aligned}
$$

while

$$
\begin{aligned}
\gamma_{xr} &= \text{logit} Pr(Y = 1 | X = x, R = r) \\
&= \log p_{x1} - \log p_{x0} + r\{\log \mu_{x1} - \log \mu_{x0}\} + \\
&\quad (1 - r)\{\log(1 - \mu_{x1}) - \log(1 - \mu_{x0})\}.
\end{aligned}
$$

The new parameterization also involves implicit components, namely $q_{00} = 1 - q_{01} - q_{10} - q_{11}$ and $\gamma_{00} = \gamma_{01} + \gamma_{10} - \gamma_{11}$. The target of inference with respect to the reparameterization is

$$
\psi \quad = \quad Pr(Y = 1) \tag{3.4}
$$

$$
= \quad \sum_{x=0}^{1} \sum_{r=0}^{1} q_{xr} \text{expit}(\gamma_{xr}). \tag{3.5}
$$

Toward computing both finite-sample posteriors and LPDs, note that the map from θ to (ϕ, λ) given above can be inverted explicitly according to:

$$
p_{xy} = q_{x0}\{\text{expit}(\gamma_{x0})\}^y\{1-\text{expit}(\gamma_{x0})\}^{1-y} + \\
q_{x1}\{\text{expit}(\gamma_{x1})\}^y\{1-\text{expit}(\gamma_{x1})\}^{1-y},
$$

and

$$
\alpha = \begin{pmatrix} 1 & 0 & 1 \\ 1 & 1 & 0 \\ 1 & 1 & 1 \end{pmatrix}^{-1} \delta,
$$

where $\delta = (\delta_{01}, \delta_{10}, \delta_{11})$, with

$$
\delta_{xy} = \text{logit} Pr(R=1|X=x, Y=y) \\
= \log \frac{q_{x1}}{q_{x0}} + y \log \frac{\text{expit}(\gamma_{x1})}{\text{expit}(\gamma_{x0})} + (1-y) \log \frac{\{1-\text{expit}(\gamma_{x1})\}}{\{1-\text{expit}(\gamma_{x0})\}}.
$$

Furthermore, while tedious, we can write down expressions for both $\partial(\phi, \lambda)/\partial\theta$ and $\partial\theta/\partial(\phi, \lambda)$. Thus we can implement the general strategies described in Chapter 2 for determining the finite-sample posterior and the LPD.

We consider inference when the prior specification is $p \sim \text{Dirichlet}(1,1,1,1)$, and the elements of $\alpha = (\alpha_0, \alpha_x, \alpha_y)$ are modelled as independent *a priori*, with mean zero normal distributions having variances σ_0^2, σ_x^2, and σ_y^2, respectively. Thus the choice of hyperparameter σ_y is pivotal. Setting $\sigma_y = 0$ corresponds to making the MAR assumption and obtaining an identified model with α_y assumed to be zero. A positive value of σ_y induces a nonidentified model, with the magnitude of plausible departures from MAR governed by the magnitude of σ_y.

To drive importance sampling for the finite-sample posterior, we need to specify a marginal convenience prior $\pi^*(\phi)$ and a conditional convenience prior $\pi^*(\lambda|\phi)$. We take the former to be "flat," specifically, $\pi^*(q, \gamma_{01}, \gamma_{11}) = \pi^*(q)\pi^*(\gamma_{01})\pi^*(\gamma_{11})$, with $q^* \sim \text{Dirichlet}(1,1,1,1)$, $\text{expit}(\gamma_{01}^*) \sim \text{Unif}(0,1)$, $\text{expit}(\gamma_{11}^*) \sim \text{Unif}(0,1)$. This results in $\pi^*(\phi|d_n)$ being both (i) tractable and (ii) proportional to the likelihood function. In particular, the components of

$$
\pi^*(\phi|d_n) = \pi^*(q|d_n)\pi^*(\gamma_{01}|d_n)\pi^*(\gamma_{11}|d_n)
$$

are

$$
\begin{aligned}
(q_{xr}^*|d_n) &\sim \text{Dirichlet}(n_{x+r}), \\
(\text{expit}(\gamma_{01}^*)|d_n) &\sim \text{Beta}(n_{011}, n_{001}), \\
(\text{expit}(\gamma_{11}^*)|d_n) &\sim \text{Beta}(n_{111}, n_{101}).
\end{aligned}
$$

To complete the algorithm, we need to specify $\pi^*(\gamma_{10}|q, \gamma_{01}, \gamma_{11})$. We know the real prior is constructed to favor parameter values "close" to the MAR assumption, so we choose this part of the convenience prior to mimic this property. Since MAR implies $\gamma_{10} = \gamma_{11}$, we take

$$\gamma_{10}^* | q, \gamma_{01}, \gamma_{11} \quad \sim \quad N(\gamma_{11}, \tau^2).$$

for some relatively small choice of τ. From here we are in business. We have a convenience prior producing a convenience posterior from which direct Monte Carlo sampling is easy to implement. And the general importance weighting scheme described in Chapter 2 allows us to make inferences with respect to the actual prior distribution.

Returning to the synthetic data in Table 3.1, we fix hyperparameters $\sigma_0 = 2$ and $\sigma_x = 2$, which correspond to relatively wide prior distributions for log odds and log odds-ratios, respectively. And we consider inferences under three values of σ_y, namely $\sigma_y = 0.1$, $\sigma_y = 0.2$, and $\sigma_y = 0.3$. The resulting point and interval estimates for the target parameter appear in Figure 3.1

To compute the bias arising from the lack of identification in this problem, we have

$$
\begin{aligned}
b_{PIM} &= E_\pi(\psi^* | \phi) - \psi \\
&= q_{00} \left[E_\pi \{ \operatorname{expit}(\gamma_{00}^*) | \phi \} - \operatorname{expit}(\gamma_{00}) \right] + \\
&\quad q_{10} \left[E_\pi \{ \operatorname{expit}(\gamma_{10}^*) | \phi \} - \operatorname{expit}(\gamma_{10}) \right] \\
&= q_{00} \left[E_\pi \{ \operatorname{expit}(\gamma_{10}^* + \gamma_{01} - \gamma_{11}) | \phi \} - \operatorname{expit}(\gamma_{10} + \gamma_{01} - \gamma_{11}) \right] + \\
&\quad q_{10} \left[E_\pi \{ \operatorname{expit}(\gamma_{10}^*) | \phi \} - \operatorname{expit}(\gamma_{10}) \right].
\end{aligned}
$$

This can be computed via one-dimensional quadrature, after applying the strategy described in Chapter 2 for determining the LPD $\pi(\gamma_{10} | q, \gamma_{01}, \gamma_{11})$ on a fine grid of points.

To contrast with the PIM bias, the IPMM bias is readily expressed in the new parameterization. The MAR assumption that $\alpha_y = 0$ induces $\gamma_{x0} = \gamma_{x1}$ for $x = 0, 1$, so that our estimator of the target will have the form

$$\hat{\psi} \quad = \quad (\hat{q}_{00} + \hat{q}_{01}) \operatorname{expit}(\hat{\gamma}_{01}) + (\hat{q}_{10} + \hat{q}_{11}) \operatorname{expit}(\hat{\gamma}_{11}),$$

producing a limiting bias

$$b_{IPMM} \quad = \quad q_{00} \{ \operatorname{expit}(\gamma_{01}) - \operatorname{expit}(\gamma_{00}) \} + q_{10} \{ \operatorname{expit}(\gamma_{11}) - \operatorname{expit}(\gamma_{10}) \}.$$

For some illustrative values of the underlying parameters, the magnitudes of the IPMM and PIM biases are plotted as a function of α_y in Figure 3.2. The hyperparameter settings for the partially identified nonignorable model are $(\sigma_0, \sigma_x, \sigma_y) = (2, 2, 0.25)$. Here the true target value is a Y prevalence of $\psi = p_{01} + p_{11} = 0.2$, while the covariate X is associated with Y according to $Pr(X = 1 | Y = 0) = p_{10}/(p_{00} + p_{10}) = 3/8$ and $Pr(X = 1 | Y = 1) = p_{11}/(p_{01} + p_{11}) = $

1/4. The four panels in the figure correspond to all combinations of $\alpha_0 = 0, 1$ and $\alpha_x = 0, 1$. Thus we consider different extents of missingness, as well as situations where missingness does and does not depend on the covariate X. Note specifically that the two combinations with $\alpha_0 = 0$ yield missingness rates of 50% (when $\alpha_x = 0$) and 42% (when $\alpha_x = 1$), in the case that $\alpha_y = 0$. These missingness rates drop to 30% and 22% for the combinations with $\alpha_0 = 1$. Given the interpretation of α_y as the log-odds ratio for $(R, Y | X)$, this choice of σ_y corresponds to postulating that the conditional odds ratio is likely between $\exp(-0.5) \approx 0.61$ and $\exp(0.5) \approx 1.65$, quantifying the notion that a very large deviation from MAR is not anticipated. We see from the figure that the two biases, while not identical, are very similar in all the settings considered. As intuitively expected, the bias is worse when the proportion of missing values is higher. The bias is largely unaffected by whether or not the missingness depends on the covariate X. ■

3.3 Reflecting Uncertainty

In Example B, we saw about the same bias price to be paid, whether the investigator pursues the IPMM route or the PIM route. Later in this chapter we will see an example where this is not always the case. First, however, we consider the indication of uncertainty that is reflected back to the investigator.

In the IPMM situation, pretty much the same story applies whether Bayesian or frequentist analysis is used. The asymptotic theory of maximum likelihood estimators in misspecified models applies (White, 1982). If the IPMM based on fixing $\theta_b = 0$ is fit to data arising from the "full" model under $\theta = \theta^\dagger$, then the estimator of θ_a will tend to

$$\tilde{\theta}_a = \operatorname{argmin}_{\theta_a} E \left[\log \left\{ \frac{\pi(d_1^\star | \theta^\dagger)}{\pi(d_1^\star | \theta^\star = (\theta_a, 0))} \right\} \right]$$

where $d_1^\star$ is a single observation arising under $\theta = \theta^\dagger$. The theory goes on to describe variability of the θ_a estimator. Let $s(\theta_a)$ be the score vector for a single observation from the IPMM model, i.e., the first derivative with respect to the parameter vector of the log density for a single observation. Let

$$A = E\left\{ s(\tilde{\theta}_a) s^T(\tilde{\theta}_a) | \theta = \theta^\dagger \right\},$$

and

$$B = E\left\{ s'(\tilde{\theta}_a) | \theta = \theta^\dagger \right\}.$$

Then, writing the maximum likelihood estimator from the IPMM based on n independent and identically distributed observations as $\hat{\theta}_{a,n}$, the result of White (1982) can be cast as

$$n^{1/2} \left\{ \hat{\theta}_{a,n} - \tilde{\theta}_a \right\} \to N\left(0, B^{-1} A B \right). \tag{3.6}$$

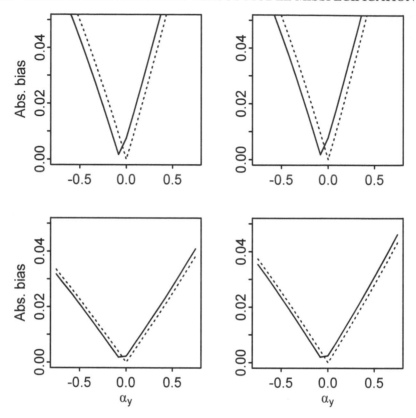

Figure 3.2 *Absolute bias of limiting point estimators as a function of the actual depar-*
ture from MAR, in Example B. The extent of departure is governed by α_y. *The dotted*
curve describes the IPMM estimator assuming MAR, while the solid curve describes
the PIM estimator using the hyperparameter setting $\sigma_y = 0.25$ *to allow possible de-*
partures from MAR. The top (bottom) panels correspond to $\alpha_0 = 0$ ($\alpha_0 = 1$). *The*
left (right) panels correspond to $\alpha_x = 0$ ($\alpha_x = 1$). *In all cases,* $(p_{00}, p_{01}, p_{10}, p_{11}) =$
$(0.5, 0.15, 0.3, 0.05)$.

This describes the $n^{1/2}$ rate at which the estimator marches toward the possibly
wrong answer $\tilde{\theta}_a$ rather than the right answer $\theta_a^{\dagger}$.

In terms of reporting a measure of uncertainty to accompany the maximum likelihood estimate of θ_a, the usual variance estimate, which does not
acknowledge the possibility of misspecification, is based on the second derivative of the log-likelihood function. Hence it will behave like $n^{-1}B$. Given that
the second derivative of the log-likelihood at the MLE will also drive the large-
sample behavior of the posterior distribution, the posterior variance of θ_a will
also behave in this manner.

At least on the likelihood estimation side, there is also the possibility of reporting a robust variance estimate motivated by the form of (3.6). The so-called "sandwich" variance estimator, which can be traced back to Huber (1967), uses empirical estimates of both A and B in order to consistently estimate the variance matrix in (3.6). This allows a properly calibrated reflection of uncertainty, but only insofar as we regard the estimator's limit as the target of inference, instead of the actual target $\tilde{g}(\theta_a, \theta_b)$. See Szpiro et al. (2010) for a Bayesian take on the sandwich estimator.

Regardless of the estimation approach adopted, reported standard errors or interval estimates will scale as $n^{-1/2}$. This lulls the investigator into a false sense of confidence, if indeed the estimator's limit differs from the actual target. Particularly, interval estimates will have frequentist coverage of the actual target tending to zero as the sample size increases. Really, in order to have any hope of correctly reflecting uncertainty, one must pursue the PIM approach. As emphasized in Chapter 2, a feature of partially identified models is that the posterior variance of the target quantity does *not* go to zero as the sample size increases, nor does the width of an interval estimate for the target. In terms of providing realistic uncertainty assessment, this is appropriate.

Example B, Continued

Continuing our discussion of estimating the prevalence of a trait which is subject to missingness, we consider interval estimates arising from the partially identified model. Since the uncertainty remaining in the large-sample limit is governed by the conditional prior density $\pi(\gamma_{10}|\gamma_{01}, \gamma_{11}, q)$, and since the target ψ is an increasing function of γ_{10} with $(\gamma_{01}, \gamma_{11}, q)$ fixed, we can determine the limiting 95% equal-tailed credible interval for ψ by plugging the 0.025 and 0.975 quantiles of $\pi(\gamma_{10}|\gamma_{01}, \gamma_{11}, q)$ into the expression for ψ.

These credible intervals, along with the limiting posterior means, are reported in Figure 3.3, for the same underlying parameter values and prior distribution considered in Figure 3.2. The salient features are as follows. In the situations with a higher proportion of missingness ($\alpha_0 = 0$), these intervals remain somewhat wide, with widths on the order of 0.1. In practical terms this is a fairly serious drawback: even with infinite data, one only learns the target prevalence to within ± 0.05. Unsurprisingly, one can learn more from the data when the missing proportion is lower ($\alpha_0 = 1$). In this case we are more in the realm of useful inference, with prevalence inferred to within about ± 0.025 in the large-sample limit.

The other main finding, albeit unsurprising, is that the quality of the limiting interval estimates is as good as the quality of the prior information supplied. Recall that the prior distribution on α_y puts its central 95% mass on the interval $\pm 2\sigma_y = (-0.5, 0.5)$. We see that when the true value of α_y is inside this interval, the limiting 95% interval on the target contains the true value. However, as α_y extends outside the prior interval, the limiting posterior interval starts to miss the target. This makes intuitive sense. If we view α_y as the parameter that is not informed by data, then we are not surprised that the quality of the inference on the target is driven by the quality of the prior information on the uninformed parameter. In fact, Gustafson (2012) gives some theoretical perspective on exactly how the compatibility of the prior on uninformed parameters with the corresponding true values dictates coverage or not for the target parameter. ■

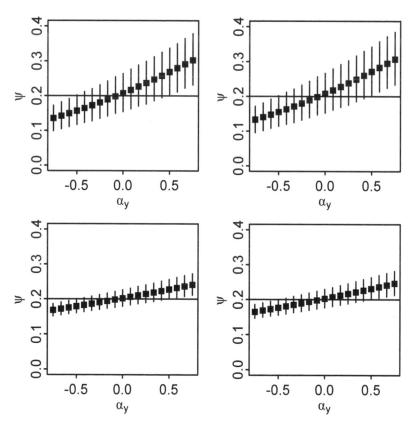

Figure 3.3 *Limiting posterior distribution on the Y-prevalence as a function of the actual departure from MAR in Example B. The extent of departure is governed by α_y. The mean and the 95% equal-tailed credible interval are depicted. The underlying parameter values and the prior distributions are as per Figure 3.2.*

3.4 A Further Example

Example C: Binary Misclassification in a Case-Control Study

As a second example of comparing IPMM and PIM strategies, consider comparing the prevalence of a binary trait across two populations, when observation of the trait is subject to nondifferential misclassification. Particularly, say the context is that of a case-control study, where the two populations correspond to healthy $(Y = 0)$ and diseased $(Y = 1)$ individuals, in which the prevalences of exposure X are $r_y = Pr(X = 1|Y = y)$, for $y = 0, 1$. However, we observe an imperfect surrogate X^* in lieu of X, with the proclivity for misclassification described by sensitivity $\gamma_N = Pr(X^* = 1|X = 1)$ and specificity $\gamma_P = Pr(X^* = 0|X = 0)$. The nondifferential assumption posits that X^* and Y are conditionally independent given X. As a target we take the log odds-ratio describing the exposure-disease association,

$$\psi = \log[r_1/(1 - r_1)] - \log[r_0/(1 - r_0)].$$

The usual case-control story pertains here. The target is defined in terms of the ratio of odds of being exposed amongst the diseased population to the odds of being exposed amongst the disease-free population. However, this odds ratio is mathematically identical to the odds of disease amongst the exposed over the odds of disease amongst the unexposed.

Our data structure is comprised of two binomial samples, from $(X^*|Y = y)$, for $y = 0, 1$. It is quickly apparent that this cannot fully inform four unknown parameters, $(r_0, r_1, \gamma_N, \gamma_P)$. Following Gustafson et al. (2001), a transparent parameterization results from taking $\phi = (\phi_0, \phi_1)$ with

$$\begin{aligned}\phi_y &= Pr(X^* = 1|Y = y) \\ &= r_y\gamma_N + (1 - r_y)(1 - \gamma_P),\end{aligned} \qquad (3.7)$$

along with $\lambda = (\gamma_N, \gamma_P)$. In general, this will also be a sticky parameterization, since (3.7) implies that $\min\{\gamma_N, 1 - \gamma_P\} \leq \min\{\phi_0, \phi_1\}$ and $\max\{\gamma_N, 1 - \gamma_P\} \geq \max\{\phi_0, \phi_1\}$.

To put the situation in focus, say a simple prior is chosen under the initial parameterization, as arises from starting with a distribution under which $(r_0, r_1, \gamma_N, \gamma_P)$ are mutually independent, but then truncating (i.e., conditioning) such that $\gamma_N + \gamma_P > 1$. This is a commonly made assumption, asserting that the classification of X into X^* is better than a random allocation not depending on X. More specifically, say the starting prior involves $r_y \sim \text{Unif}(0, 1)$ for $y = 0, 1$, $\gamma_N \sim \text{Beta}(a_N, b_N)$, $\gamma_P \sim \text{Beta}(a_P, b_P)$. This corresponds to an investigator who is unable or unwilling to input substantive prior information about exposure prevalences, but can represent beliefs about the quality of the exposure classification, through appropriate choices of hyperparameters for the Beta prior distributions on sensitivity and specificity.

Before proceeding further with the analysis via this partially identified model, consider the investigator who instead chooses the identified but possibly misspecified modelling route, by treating guessed values of sensitivity and specificity as known. Expressed in the transparent parameterization, the target is

$$\psi = \log(\phi_1 + \gamma_P - 1) - \log(\gamma_N - \phi_1) - \\ \log(\phi_0 + \gamma_P - 1) + \log(\gamma_N - \phi_0). \tag{3.8}$$

Thus the limit of the IPMM estimator will be of the form (3.8), supplied with the correct values of (ϕ_0, ϕ_1), but possibly erroneous guesses, which we denote as $(\tilde{\gamma}_N, \tilde{\gamma}_P)$, in place of the actual sensitivity and specificity (γ_N, γ_P).

Returning to the investigator working with the PIM, prior distributions can be assigned to (γ_N, γ_P) which are centered at the guessed values $(\tilde{\gamma}_N, \tilde{\gamma}_P)$, while acknowledging the uncertainty in the guesses. To give a firm example, say the guessed values are $(\tilde{\gamma}_N, \tilde{\gamma}_P) = (0.75, 0.9)$. However, the investigator is only confident that each actual value is within ± 0.05 of the guess. Consequently, priors based on $(a_N, b_N) = (214.5, 71.5)$ and $(a_P, b_P) = (119.7, 13.3)$ are selected. These hyperparameters are chosen to give $E(\gamma_N^\star) = \tilde{\gamma}_N$ and $Pr(\gamma_N^\star \in \tilde{\gamma}_N \pm 0.05) = 0.95$ for sensitivity, and similarly $E(\gamma_P^\star) = \tilde{\gamma}_P$ and $Pr(\gamma_P^\star \in \tilde{\gamma}_P \pm 0.05) = 0.95$ for specificity. It is worth noting that these are indeed highly informative prior distributions. For instance, with respect to binomial updating, the sum of the two Beta hyperparameters can be regarded as an effective sample size, i.e., the strength of the prior on the sensitivity corresponds to observation of apparent exposure status for $214.5 + 71.5 = 285$ truly exposed subjects, while the strength of the prior on specificity corresponds to observation of apparent exposure status for $119.7 + 13.3 = 133$ truly unexposed subjects. While this can be regarded as a very considerable degree of *a priori* knowledge, we must remember it assumes much less than the IPMM route of taking γ_N and γ_P to be known.

Following Gustafson et al. (2001), the limiting posterior distribution is characterized by a point-mass distribution at the true values of (ϕ_0, ϕ_1) combined with the conditional prior distribution of $(\gamma_N, \gamma_P | \phi_0, \phi_1)$. This conditional distribution has a density of the form

$$\pi(\gamma_N, \gamma_P | \phi_0, \phi_1) \propto (\gamma_N + \gamma_P - 1)^{-2} \pi(\gamma_N; a_N, b_N) \pi(\gamma_P; a_P, b_P) \times \\ I\{\gamma_N > \max(\phi_0, \phi_1), \gamma_P > 1 - \min(\phi_0, \phi_1)\}. \tag{3.9}$$

Thus the limiting posterior mean of the target is the mean of (3.8) with respect to the distribution described by (3.9), with the correct values of (ϕ_0, ϕ_1) supplied.

The form of (3.9) is simple enough that we do not need to resort to Monte Carlo methods to compute properties of the LPD. Rather, we simply use two-dimensional numerical quadrature. Particularly, we can use quantiles of the prior distributions for γ_N and γ_P as evaluation points. To be clear on this, for a quantity of interest $s(\gamma_N, \gamma_P)$ we can write

$$E_\pi\{s(\gamma_N^\star, \gamma_P^\star)|\phi\} = \frac{E_\pi\left\{s(\gamma_N^\star, \gamma_P^\star)(\gamma_N^\star + \gamma_P^\star - 1)^{-2}I_{R(\phi)}(\gamma_N^\star, \gamma_P^\star)\right\}}{E_\pi\left\{(\gamma_N^\star + \gamma_P^\star - 1)^{-2}I_{R(\phi)}(\gamma_N^\star, \gamma_P^\star)\right\}}(3.10)$$

Then a convenient quadrature scheme for both the numerator and denominator expectations arises by transforming the prior distributions for γ_N and γ_P to uniform distributions. Explicitly, let $U_N^\star$ and $U_P^\star$ have independent $\text{Unif}(0,1)$ distributions, and take $\gamma_N^\star = F_\beta^{-1}(U_N^\star; a_N, b_N)$ and $\gamma_P^\star = F_\beta^{-1}(U_P^\star; a_P, b_P)$, where $F_\beta(\bullet; a, b)$ is the $\text{Beta}(a, b)$ distribution function. Then both expectations in (3.10) can be reexpressed as expectations with respect to $(U_N^\star, U_P^\star)$. In turn, these can be computed numerically via evaluation on an equidistant grid of points in the unit square.

In the scenario of true exposure prevalences $(r_0, r_1) = (0.06, 0.09)$, the biases b_{IPMM} and b_{PIM} are computed for a range of true values for (γ_N, γ_P), and reported in Figure 3.4. Note that the true value of the target is $\psi = \log 1.55$, corresponding to a sizeable exposure-disease association. A first point to make is that some true values of (γ_N, γ_P), even within the guessed ranges of $\tilde{\gamma}_N \pm 0.05$, $\tilde{\gamma}_P \pm 0.05$, cause b_{IPMM} to "blow-up." That is, supplying these values in (3.8), along with correct values of (ϕ_0, ϕ_1), yields nonsensical estimates in which r_0 and/or r_1 are estimated to be outside the unit interval. Particularly, this occurs when the true value of specificity is near the upper end of the guessed range. Commensurately, the IPMM bias gets very large in magnitude as the true value of specificity increases toward the blow-up case. In contrast, the PIM bias is much better behaved. It is somewhat asymmetric, with specificity values above the guess inducing more bias than values the same distance below the guess. Note as well that both b_{IPMM} and b_{PIM} are largely unaffected by γ_N as γ_P stays fixed. This reflects that for a rare exposure, good information about specificity is more crucial than good information about sensitivity, simply because the sample contains far more truly unexposed subjects than truly exposed subjects.

Figure 3.5 gives the results of redoing the bias comparison in the situation of higher exposure prevalences $(r_0, r_1) = (0.15, 0.21)$. Note that this corresponds to about the same odds ratio as before, i.e., now $\psi = \log 1.51$. Similarly, Figure 3.6 corresponds to $(r_0, r_1) = (0.35, 0.45)$, with $\psi = \log 1.52$. As we move to higher exposure prevalences, we see that (i) the IPMM and PIM biases become very close to one another, (ii) these biases both become smaller, and (iii) the discrepancy between the guessed and actual values of γ_N become more important.

Turning to the reflection of uncertainty, we can report on the magnitude of posterior uncertainty and the calibration of the posterior distribution as follows. In the case that $(r_0, r_1) = (0.08, 0.12)$, again giving an odds ratio near 1.5, Figure 3.7 displays the limiting posterior standard deviation of the target

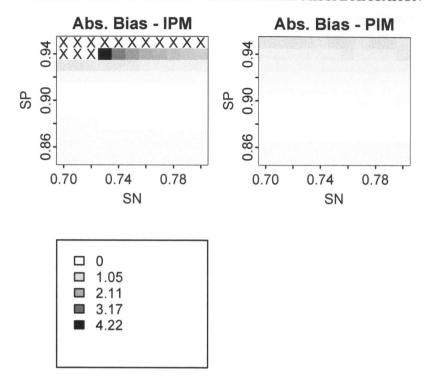

Figure 3.4 *Limiting absolute bias for estimating the log odds-ratio in Example C, as a function of the true sensitivity and specificity, when $(r_0, r_1) = (0.06, 0.09)$. In the case of the IPMM bias, 'X' indicates a situation where the estimator limit is not well defined.*

ψ, for various true values of (γ_P, γ_N). This is seen to vary with (γ_P, γ_N) to a surprisingly large extent. The posterior quantile at which the true target value lies is also reported. Note that the compatibility of the guessed and true values of sensitivity is largely irrelevant, with the calibration of the answer driven by the prior on specificity. That is, if the true value of γ_P lies at the α quantile of the prior on γ_P, then the true value of ψ is seen to lie in the rough vicinity of the $1 - \alpha$ quantile of the limiting posterior distribution.

Figure 3.7 also reports on the extent to which the IPMM analysis under-reports uncertainty about the target. In the present situation we do not need the full generality of (3.6). Rather, we proceed as follows. We know that unless the guessed values of sensitivity and specificity are correct, the confidence interval for the target ψ will shrink down to the wrong point as the sample size n increases. We assume the balanced case in which n controls and n cases are sampled, and write the target (3.8) as $\psi = g_\gamma(\phi)$, which gets estimated as $\hat{\psi} = g_{\tilde{\gamma}}(\hat{\phi})$. Thus the nominal $(1 - \alpha)$ confidence interval for the target will behave

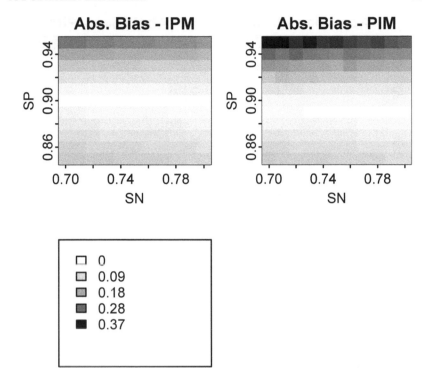

Figure 3.5 *Limiting absolute bias for estimating the log odds-ratio in Example C, as a function of the true sensitivity and specificity, when* $(r_0, r_1) = (0.15, 0.21)$.

like $g_{\tilde{\phi}}(\hat{\phi}) \pm z_{\alpha/2} n^{-1/2} \sigma(\hat{\phi})$, where

$$\sigma(\phi) = \left[\{g'_{\tilde{\gamma}}(\phi)\}^T I^{-1}(\phi) \{g'_{\tilde{\gamma}}(\phi)\} \right]^{1/2},$$

and $z_{\alpha/2}$ is the $1\text{-}\alpha/2$ quantile of the standard normal distribution. The information matrix $I(\phi)$ in this problem is simply diagonal, with entries $\phi_i^{-1}(1 - \phi_i)^{-1}$, for $i = 0, 1$. The probability that the interval fails to cover the true target is thus approximately $\Phi(n^{1/2}|g_{\tilde{\gamma}}(\phi) - g_{\gamma}(\phi)|/\sigma(\phi) - z_{\alpha/2})$, where $\Phi(\bullet)$ is the standard normal distribution function. Consequently, the sample size at which the actual coverage drops to $1 - \alpha^*$ is given approximately as

$$n^* \quad - \quad \left(\frac{|z_{\alpha^*/2} - z_{\alpha/2}|\sigma(\phi)}{|g_{\gamma}(\phi) - g_{\tilde{\gamma}}(\phi)|} \right)^2.$$

Figure 3.7 shows how n^* varies with the underlying values of γ_N and γ_P. We see it is the discrepancy between guessed and true values of specificity, rather

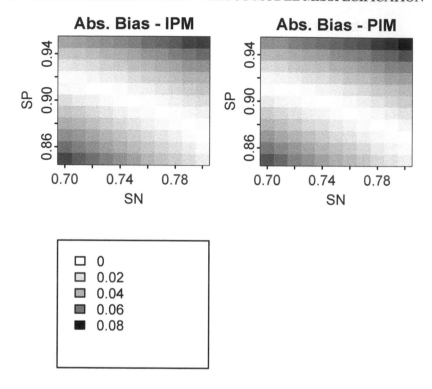

Figure 3.6 *Limiting absolute bias for estimating the log odds-ratio in Example C, as a function of the true sensitivity and specificity, when* $(r_0, r_1) = (0.35, 0.45)$.

than sensitivity, that govern the under-reporting of uncertainty. Unsurprisingly, a larger discrepancy implies that undercoverage occurs at a smaller sample size.

As a second example of reflecting uncertainty in this problem, Figure 3.8 describes the situation for higher exposure prevalences of $(r_0, r_1) = (0.23, 0.31)$. The findings are qualitatively very similar to those in Figure 3.7, though with the higher exposure prevalences we start to see the true value of sensitivity play a small role.

To round out this example, we consider finite-sample inference. Let n_{ab} be the number of subjects with $(Y = a, X^* = b)$, so that n_{0+} and n_{1+} are the control and case sample sizes, respectively. We will employ the importance sampling strategy from Chapter 2. The marginal convenience prior $\pi^*(\phi_0, \phi_1)$ is taken as the uniform distribution on $(0, 1)^2$. To obtain the correct support for the convenience posterior, the conditional convenience prior is based on truncated Beta distributions. Letting $f_\beta(\bullet; a, b)$ denote the Beta(a, b) density function, and recalling that $F_\beta(\bullet; a, b)$ denotes the Beta(a, b) distribution function, we

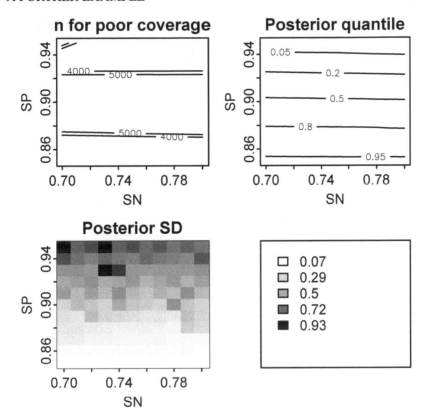

Figure 3.7 *Reflection of uncertainty as the true sensitivity and specificity vary in Example C, when $(r_0, r_1) = (0.08, 0.12)$. The top-left panel gives the sample size n at which the 95% confidence interval from the IPMM model has only 80% coverage. The top-right panel describes the whereabouts of the true log odds-ratio in the limiting posterior distribution, in terms of the quantile at which the true value lies. The bottom-left panel gives the limiting posterior standard deviation of the log odds-ratio.*

take

$$\pi^*(\gamma_N|\phi) = \frac{f_\beta(\gamma_N; a_N, b_N)I_{(\max\{\phi_0, \phi_1\}, 1)}(\gamma_N)}{1 - F_\beta(\max\{\phi_0, \phi_1\}; a_N, b_N)}$$

and

$$\pi^*(\gamma_P|\phi) = \frac{f_\beta(\gamma_P; a_P, b_P)I_{(1-\min\{\phi_0, \phi_1\}, 1)}(\gamma_P)}{1 - F_\beta(1 - \min\{\phi_0, \phi_1\}; a_P, b_P)}.$$

With this specification, direct Monte Carlo sampling from the convenience posterior distribution is easy. We have $\pi^*(\phi|d_n)$ characterized by $(\phi_0^*|d_n) \sim$

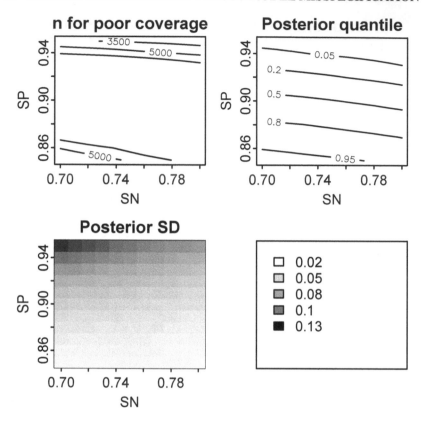

Figure 3.8 *Reflection of uncertainty as the true sensitivity and specificity vary in Example C, when* $(r_0, r_1) = (0.23, 0.31)$. *The format is as per Figure 3.7.*

Beta$(1+n_{01}, 1+n_{00})$ independently of $(\phi_1^{\star}|d_n) \sim$ Beta$(1+n_{11}, 1+n_{10})$. Moreover, Monte Carlo sampling from the truncated Beta distributions in $\pi^*(\gamma|\phi)$ is easily coded by considering the probability integral transform, so that sampling from truncated uniform distributions (which themselves are uniform) is all that is required. The importance weights end up with a simple form,

$$
\begin{aligned}
w(\phi_0, \phi_1, \gamma_N, \gamma_P) \quad \propto \quad & [1 - F_\beta(\max\{\phi_0, \phi_1\}; a_N, b_N)] \times \\
& [1 - F_\beta(1 - \min\{\phi_0, \phi_1\}; a_P, b_P)] \times \\
& (\gamma_N + \gamma_P - 1)^{-2}.
\end{aligned}
$$

With a computational approach in hand, we display the progression with sample size of the marginal posterior distribution of ψ, for some synthetic data-streams. Figure 3.9 gives results for three independently generated data-streams, each making stops at $n_{i+} = 100$, $n_{i+} = 400$, and $n_{i+} = 1600$. These data are generated under $(\phi_0, \phi_1) = (0.10, 0.15)$, while the prior distribution is based on $(a_N, b_N) = (a_P, b_P) = (135, 15)$. This specification corresponds to a best guess of 90% for the sensitivity γ_P and 90% for the specificity γ_N, with an "effective sample size" of 150. That is, the prior strength corresponds to observing X^* for 150 subjects known to be unexposed $(X = 0)$ and 150 subjects known to be exposed $(X = 1)$. As a more direct quantification of prior uncertainty, the 95% equal-tailed interval for the Beta(135,15) distribution is $(0.847, 0.942)$. Note that here we have deliberately chosen a scenario whereby the data can "cut into" the prior distribution. To explain, in the large-sample limit we learn that $\gamma_P > 1 - \min\{\phi_0, \phi_1\} = 0.9$, hence there is considerable scope for prior-to-posterior updating of γ_P.

The tri-interval plots in Figure 3.9 tell a familiar tail of diminishing returns. In moving from $n = 100$ to $n = 400$ we see some posterior narrowing, albeit not by the factor of two that would arise in the identified model case. Then, however, we see only marginal improvement from $n = 400$ to $n = 1600$, by which point we have almost attained the narrowness of the LPD. It also must be pointed out that we are in a setting where the LPD itself is quite uncertain about the magnitude of the (X, Y) association, given its width on the log odds-ratio scale.

A second example of the progression with sample size is given in Figure 3.10. All the settings are as above, except now the parameters underlying the data generation are $(\phi_0, \phi_1) = (0.15, 0.20)$. The impact of this change is that the identification region bound of $\gamma_P > 1 - \min\{\phi_0, \phi_1\} = 0.85$ now takes a much "smaller bite" out of the prior distribution for γ_P. That is, there is much less scope for prior-to-posterior updating of γ_P in this setting. Nonetheless, the LPD happens to be much narrower in this setting than in the previous one, by more than a factor of two in terms of 95% HPD interval length. A partial explanation for this is that generally more common exposures lead to more precise log odds-ratio estimation. For instance, setting aside misclassification concerns, the standard log odds-ratio estimator for the (X^*, Y) association has variance behaving as $\{n_0 \phi_0 (1 - \phi_0)\}^{-1} + \{n_1 \phi_1 (1 - \phi_1)\}^{-1}$. This implies about a 20% reduction in estimator standard deviation upon moving from the first scenario to the second. Of course this leaves much of the large reduction in LPD width unexplained. This is in keeping with a general theme of partially identified models: the performance of estimators can vary quite dramatically as the underlying true parameter values change, to an extent not seen typically in identified settings. Having said this, Figures 3.9 and 3.10 also show a sense in which the two scenarios induce the same behavior. Relative to the LPD, the rate at which the posterior narrows with respect to n is quite similar to across the two settings.

Finally, we take the first data-stream in Figure 3.9 and the first data-stream in Figure 3.10, and consider inference about the specificity, γ_P. This is portrayed in Figure 3.11, via both the progression with sample size for the

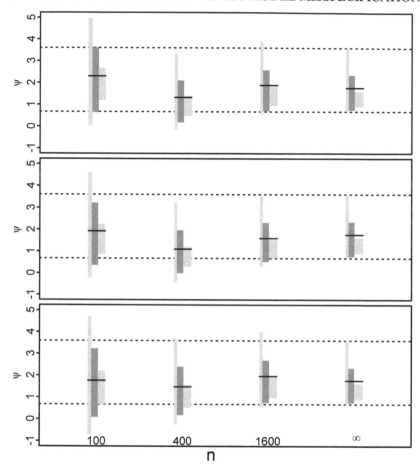

Figure 3.9 *Finite sample evolution of the posterior distribution of* ψ *in Example C. Three synthetic data-streams are simulated under* $(\phi_0, \phi_1) = (0.10, 0.15)$. *The prior specification is based on* $(a_N, b_N) = (a_P, b_P) = (135, 15)$. *All the posteriors (finite-sample and limiting) were computed via a Monte Carlo sample of size 50,000. The smallest effective sample size is 17,500 in the* $n = 100$ *instances, and* $42,200$ *in the other instances. The dotted horizontal reference lines give the 95% HPD interval for the LPD, to help visualize the magnitude of sampling variability across the three replicated data-streams.*

marginal posterior distribution of γ_P and a comparison of the prior and limiting posterior distributions of γ_P. As expected, in the first setting the data do "take a bite" out of the prior distribution, such that appreciable updating of γ_P occurs. Conversely, in the second setting the LPD for γ_P is extremely similar to the prior distribution, and there is no appreciable narrowing with sample size.

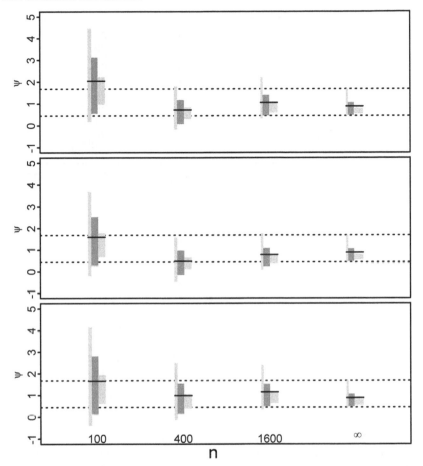

Figure 3.10 *Finite sample evolution of the posterior distribution of ψ in Example C. Three synthetic data-streams are simulated under $(\phi_0, \phi_1) = (0.15, 0.20)$. The prior specification is based on $(a_N, b_N) = (a_P, b_P) = (135, 15)$. All the posteriors (finite-sample and limiting) were computed via a Monte Carlo sample of size 50,000, The smallest effective sample size is 37,700 in the $n = 100$ instances, and 49,200 in the other instances. The dotted horizontal reference lines give the 95% HPD interval for the LPD, to help see the magnitude of sampling variability across the three replicated data-streams.*

This provides an excellent example of a common PIM phenomenon. Depending on where in the parameter space the true parameter values lie, there could be appreciable updating about a given parameter upon receipt of data, or there could be virtually no updating. ∎

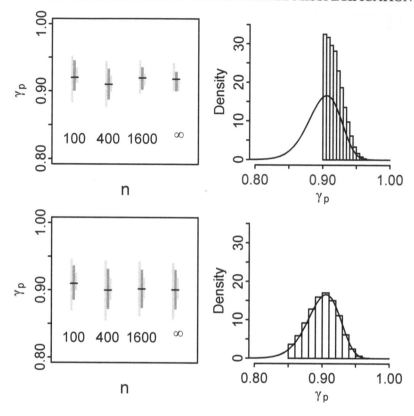

Figure 3.11 *Posterior distribution on specificity in Example C. The top panels correspond to the first data-stream in Figure 3.9 with $(\phi_0, \phi_1) = (0.10, 0.15)$, and the bottom panels correspond to the first data-stream in Figure 3.10 with $(\phi_0, \phi_1) = (0.15, 0.20)$. The left panels give the posterior marginal on γ_P as a function of n. The right panels compare the LPD on γ_P (histogram) to the prior distribution (smooth curve).*

3.5   Other Investigations of PIM versus IPMM

There are other direct comparisons of the PIM and IPMM biases in the literature. For instance, Gustafson and Greenland (2006) consider the context of regressing an outcome variable on a "short list" of predictors, each of which is a deterministic function of variables on a "long list" of predictors. The motivating example involves the long list being person-level intakes of many diet items, as ascertained from a questionnaire. The short list is comprised of intakes of some nutrients, each of which is calculated as a linear combination of diet item intakes. In this problem, θ_a and θ_b correspond to regression coefficients for the short-list predictors and the long-list predictors, respectively, in a regression of the outcome on *all* the predictors. Common practice in nutritional epidemiology settings would be to simply regress the outcome on the nutrients only, which corresponds to inferring θ_a under the assumption that $\theta_b = 0$. This corresponds to inference under an identified model. However, it also corresponds to a hard-to-justify assumption that the only way the food items influence the outcome is via the nutrients. If we weaken this assumption and treat (θ_a, θ_b) as jointly unknown, we are likely on firmer scientific ground. Unfortunately, however, we are also on partially identified ground. There are exact colinearities in that the nutrient variables are linear combinations of the diet item variables. Therefore, the model lacks identification. Some regularization can be introduced, in the way of a prior distribution which postulates that large effects of diet items beyond their impact via nutrients is unlikely. Then we have a comparison exactly of the form of (3.2) versus (3.1). Gustafson and Greenland (2006) are indeed able to show that the two biases behave very similarly when θ_b is very small in magnitude, but as the diet item coefficients grow, the bias due to model misspecification grows faster than the bias due to partial identification. Thus in this example honesty is the best policy. If we cannot justify the assumption that the diet items have no direct effect on the outcome, then we are better off incurring the PIM bias with statistical modelling which reflects this, rather than the IPMM bias based on optimistically assuming there are no direct effects of diet items that bypass the nutrient variables.

Another example of comparing the PIM and IPMM biases is given in Gustafson (2007). Here the context is that of using an *instrumental variable* to help form inferences about the relationship between an outcome and an exposure, when the exposure cannot be measured well. This requires that the variable identified as the instrument be associated with the exposure but have no direct effect on the outcome beyond an indirect effect via exposure. In the measurement error context, having one unbiased surrogate for exposure plus an instrument is a weaker assumption than having two unbiased surrogates, yet either serves to render consistent estimation of the exposure-disease association. On the downside, however, the assumption that the instrument has no direct effect on the outcome beyond an indirect effect via exposure is not empirically testable, since the true exposure is unobserved. In the context of normal linear models, Gustafson (2007) takes θ_b as the regression coefficient for the instrument in a model for the outcome given exposure and instrument, while θ_a includes all other parameters, including those in a model for the surrogate exposure given the true exposure, and those in a model for the true exposure given the instrument. Thus the comparison between (3.1) and (3.2) is again relevant. The IPMM bias is zero when $\theta_b = 0$, but it transpires that as θ_b departs from zero, the IPMM bias quickly becomes larger in magnitude than the PIM bias. Thus again it is a case of honesty in modelling being the best policy. Some further remarks on Gustafson (2007) appear later in Chapter 7, Section 7.3.

Chapter 4

Further Examples: Models Involving Misclassification

4.1 Binary to Trinary Misclassification

In Example C of Chapter 3 we considered the problem of inferring the association between a binary X and a binary Y, when the available data are observations of (X^*, Y) rather than (X, Y). Recall that in this context X^*, which is also binary, is regarded as a "noisy surrogate" for X. Moreover, the quality of the surrogate is quantified by its sensitivity, $Pr(X^* = 1 | X = 1)$, and specificity, $Pr(X^* = 0 | X = 0)$. Also recall that the assumption of *nondifferential* misclassification may be warranted, whereby conditional independence between X^* and Y given X is assumed. Often in a biostatistical context, X indicates absence or presence of an exposure and Y indicates disease status. Then nondifferentiality corresponds to the imperfect measurement of exposure being completely blind to disease status.

Example D: Classification with a "Maybe" Category

Here we branch out from Example C with a version of this problem where X and Y are still binary, but now X^* is trinary. This could arise in an epidemiological context, particularly when the exposure measurement involves expert judgment. In an occupational epidemiology study, for instance, an occupational hygienist might be tasked with determining the exposure status of workers within a cohort. Even though the true exposure is well defined in terms of absence ($X = 0$) or presence ($X = 1$), based on the imperfect information available for a given subject, the assessor could report the subject as unlikely to be exposed ($X^* = 0$), perhaps exposed ($X^* = 1$), or likely exposed ($X^* = 2$). Commensurately, sensitivity and specificity are generalized to classification probabilities $p_{ij} = Pr(X^* = j | X = i)$, for $i = 0, 1$ and $j = 0, 1, 2$. Again we focus on the nondifferential version of the problem, where conditional independence of X^* and Y given X is assumed.

We can take the initial scientific parameterization for this problem as

$$\theta = (r_0, r_1, p_{00}, p_{02}, p_{10}, p_{12}), \qquad (4.1)$$

where, as per Example C, $r_i = Pr(X = 1|Y = i)$. Note that $p_{i1} = 1 - p_{i0} - p_{i2}$ is defined implicity. In fact choosing the "middle" probabilities as those to omit from (4.1) is actually quite deliberate, for reasons soon made apparent. Given the nondifferentiality assumption, θ completely describes the distribution of $(X, X^*|Y)$, and in turn the observable distribution of $(X^*|Y)$. Indeed, we assume the available data take the form of two multinomial observations, of size n_{0+} from $(X^*|Y = 0)$ and size n_{1+} from $(X^*|Y = 1)$. These correspond to the control and case samples in a case-control study, and we can use n_{yc} to denote the number of subjects with $(Y = y, X^* = c)$, for $y = 0, 1$, $c = 0, 1, 2$.

Transparent Reparameterization

Following Wang et al. (2012), a transparent parameterization for this problem arises by taking $\phi = (q_{00}, q_{02}, q_{10}, q_{02})$ and $\lambda = (z_0, z_1)$, where

$$
\begin{aligned}
q_{ij} &= Pr(X^* = j|Y = i) \\
&= Pr(X = 0|Y = i)Pr(X^* = j|X = 0) + \\
&\quad Pr(X = 1|Y = i)Pr(X^* = j|X = 1) \\
&= (1 - r_i)p_{0j} + r_i p_{1j},
\end{aligned}
$$

while

$$
\begin{aligned}
z_0 &= r_0/(r_1 - r_0) \\
z_1 &= (1 - r_1)/(r_1 - r_0).
\end{aligned}
$$

Note that again the probabilities corresponding to the middle level of X^* are omitted from ϕ. Clearly the distribution of the observable data for $(X^*|Y)$ depends on θ only through ϕ. It is also straightforward to verify that the map from θ to (ϕ, λ) is invertible, according to

$$
\begin{aligned}
p_{0j} &= q_{0j} + z_0(q_{0j} - q_{1j}) \\
p_{1j} &= q_{1j} + z_1(q_{1j} - q_{0j}) \\
r_0 &= z_0/(1 + z_0 + z_1) \\
r_1 &= (1 + z_0)/(1 + z_0 + z_1).
\end{aligned}
$$

The algebraic expressions above become more penetrable upon taking a geometric view of the problem. Before getting to this, however, we discuss possible forms of prior knowledge about the classification probabilities p_{ij}. Recall that in Example C we made the weak assumption that the sum of sensitivity and specificity exceeds one. This is the "classification is better than random" assumption, since a Bernoulli(s) random variable *independent* of X will have sensitivity plus specificity of $s + (1 - s) = 1$ as a surrogate for X. A natural extension to the present situation would be the assumption that as binary surrogates for X *both* $I\{X^* > 0\}$ and $I\{X^* > 1\}$ are better than random. That is, the surrogate formed from collapsing from three categories to two carries some information about X, whether the "maybe" group is combined with the "unlikely" group, or with the "likely" group. Formally, we will say that the classification probabilities satisfy the *basic assumption* provided $p_{00} > p_{10}$ (implying $p_{01} + p_{02} < p_{11} + p_{12}$) *and* $p_{12} > p_{02}$ (implying $p_{10} + p_{11} < p_{00} + p_{01}$). And we shall only consider prior distributions assigning all their weight to classification probabilities satisfying the basic assumption.

As we have seen in earlier chapters, in partially identified contexts it is often of interest to examine how posterior inferences improve if strong prior assumptions can be invoked. A stronger notion of "reasonably behaving" classification probabilities would be that of monotonicity, whereby $p_{00} > p_{01} > p_{02}$ and $p_{10} < p_{11} < p_{12}$. This state of affairs can be summarized as stating that worse classifications are less likely, for both truly unexposed subjects and truly exposed subjects. The monotonicity assumption is easily seen to imply the basic assumption. In moving from the basic assumption to the monotonicity assumption then, we can think of moving to a prior distribution with smaller support.

Geometric Interpretation

Now we are well positioned to discuss the geometry of the situation. Think of a distribution on X^* as a point (a, b) in the unit square, with $a = Pr(X^* = 2)$ on the horizontal axis and $b = Pr(X^* = 0)$ on the vertical axis. Immediately we see that a point corresponds to a legitimate distribution if and only if it lies in the lower-left triangle of the square, so that $Pr(X^* = 0) + Pr(X^* = 2) \leq 1$. Moreover, by taking this view we can visualize both the basic and monotonicity assumptions. Let $\tilde{p}_i = (p_{i2}, p_{i0})$, so that $\tilde{p}_i$ is the "visualized vector" version of $p_i = (p_{i0}, p_{i1}, p_{i2})$, for $i = 0, 1$. Moreover, let $\mathbb{T}$ denote the lower-left triangle of the unit square, so that $\tilde{p}_i \in \mathbb{T}$. Then the basic assumption can be expressed as $(\tilde{p}_0, \tilde{p}_1) \in \mathbb{P}_B$, where $\mathbb{P}_B$ is the subset of $\mathbb{T} \times \mathbb{T}$ for which $\tilde{p}_1$ lies both below and to the right of $\tilde{p}_0$. Or, more colloquially, $\tilde{p}_1$ is southeast of $\tilde{p}_0$. Similarly, the monotonicity assumption is expressed as $(\tilde{p}_0, \tilde{p}_1) \in \mathbb{P}_M = \mathbb{T}_0 \times \mathbb{T}_1$, where $\mathbb{T}_0$ and $\mathbb{T}_1$ are disjoint triangular subsets of $\mathbb{T}$, as depicted in Figure 4.1.

Again using the tilde notation, such that $\tilde{q}_i$ is the vector version of $q_i = (q_{i0}, q_{i1}, q_{i2})$, we can gain insight into the geometry of the problem. By construction, $\tilde{q}_0$ and $\tilde{q}_1$ must fall on the line segment joining $\tilde{p}_0$ and $\tilde{p}_1$. And of course the data speak directly to the values of $(\tilde{q}_0, \tilde{q}_1)$ through the likelihood function, such that these become known in the large-sample limit. Henceforth we refer to the line passing through both $\tilde{q}_0$ and $\tilde{q}_1$ as "the connecting line." And we note that the basic assumption, $(\tilde{p}_0, \tilde{p}_1) \in \mathbb{P}_B$, guarantees that the connecting line will have negative slope. Therefore, the indirect information be-

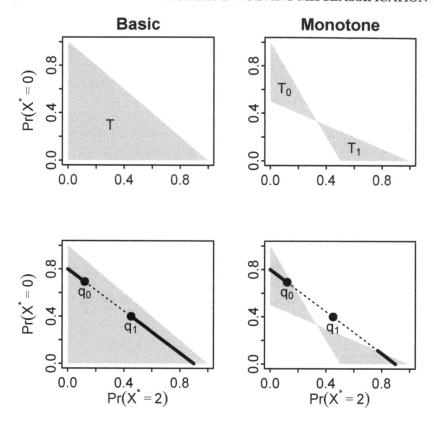

Figure 4.1 *Geometric view of identification regions in Example D. The upper panels simply illustrate the prior regions under the basic assumption (left panel) and the monotonicity assumption (right panel). For given q, the identification regions for $\tilde{p}_0$ and $\tilde{p}_1$ are given by the thicker black line segments. Note that the particular values for q are such that the identification region for p_0 is the same under the basic and monotonicity assumptions, whereas the identification region for p_1 is much reduced upon making the stronger monotonicity assumption.*

coming available in the large-sample limit is that $\tilde{p}_0$ must lie somewhere on the connecting line, between the the more northwesterly of $\tilde{q}_0$ and $\tilde{q}_1$ and the northwestern boundary of $\mathbb{T}$. Similarly $\tilde{p}_1$ must lie on the line somewhere between the most southeasterly of the two points and the southeastern boundary of $\mathbb{T}$. This notion is illustrated in the left panels of Figure 4.1.

To relate the geometry back to the algebraic expressions, it is immediate that for given values of $\tilde{q}_i$ that are compatible with the basic assumption (i.e., the connecting line has negative slope), the possible values of $\tilde{p}_i$ correspond to a finite rectangular region of (z_0, z_1) values. Implicit here is that our transparent parameterization (ϕ, λ) is a sticky parameterization. When making only the basic assumption, we write the rectangular region as $(z_0, z_1) \in \mathbb{Z}_B(q)$, such that $c_i^{(B)} \leq z_i \leq d_i^{(B)}$, for $i = 0, 1$. In the case that q_1 is southeast of q_0 (as illustrated in Figure 4.1), we have that $c_0^{(B)} = c_1^{(B)} = 0$, while $d_0^{(B)}$ is the value of z_0 which maps $\tilde{p}_0$ onto the boundary of $\mathbb{T}$ northwest of $\tilde{q}_0$ (intersecting either the line $a = 0$ or the line $b = 1 - a$, depending on the nature of the connecting line). Similarly, $d_1^{(B)}$ is the value of z_1 for which $\tilde{p}_1$ hits the boundary of $\mathbb{T}$ to the southeast of $\tilde{q}_1$. Explicit algebraic forms for $d_i^{(B)}$ are cumbersome to write down; however, the interested reader can find them embedded in the online code. The same arguments apply in the other situation that $\tilde{q}_1$ is northwest of $\tilde{q}_0$, except now $d_i^{(B)} = -1$, for $i = 0, 1$, with $c_i^{(B)}$ determined by the connecting line hitting the boundary of $\mathbb{T}$. Again, algebraic details are embedded in the online code. Toward elucidating the limiting posterior distribution then, provided the prior distribution on $\theta = (r_0, r_1, p)$ is fully supported on $(0, 1)^2 \times \mathbb{P}_B$, the prior conditional distribution of $(z|q)$, which is equivalently the limiting posterior distribution, will be supported on $\mathbb{Z}_B(q)$. We also note from the form of the map between (r_0, r_1) and (z_0, z_1) that the rectangular identification region for z is equivalently a quadrilateral identification region for r.

The same general approach applies when the monotonicity assumption is invoked. Again intersecting the prior region with the "exterior" segments of the connecting line reveals the identification region, as encoded by the values of z which are compatible with q, denoted $\mathbb{Z}_M(q)$. As a preliminary, note that by definition if $\tilde{p} \in \mathbb{P}_M$, then $\tilde{q}$ must spawn a connecting line that intersects $a = 0$ between $b = 1/2$ and $b = 1$, and intersects $b = 0$ between $a = 1/2$ and $a = 1$. We say such a line is compatible with monotonicity. It is visually apparent that a line not having this property cannot intersect both $\mathbb{T}_0$ and $\mathbb{T}_1$, which would contradict $\tilde{p} \in \mathbb{P}_M$. As a brief further thought in this direction, for some values of θ for which $\tilde{p} \in \mathbb{P}_B \setminus \mathbb{P}_M$, monotonicity is empirically falsifiable, precisely because the resulting connecting line is not compatible with monotonicity. However, it is also visually clear there are other values of θ with $\tilde{p} \in \mathbb{P}_B \setminus \mathbb{P}_M$ for which the connecting line is compatible, hence monotonicity is not empirically falsifiable in such cases.

To understand $\mathbb{Z}_M(q)$, note first that under some circumstances we will have $\mathbb{Z}_M(q) = \mathbb{Z}_B(q)$. For instance, say $\tilde{q}_1$ is southeast of $\tilde{q}_0$. Should it be that $\tilde{q}_0 \in \mathbb{T}_0$ and $\tilde{q}_1 \in \mathbb{T}_1$, then the segments of the connecting line to the northwest of $\tilde{q}_0$ and to the southeast of $\tilde{q}_1$ are wholly within the prior region. Hence $\mathbb{Z}_M(q) = \mathbb{Z}_B(q)$. On the other hand, consider the situation in the lower-right panel of Figure 4.1. Since $\tilde{q}_0 \in \mathbb{T}_0$, it is immediate that $c_0^{(M)}(q) = c_0^{(B)}(q) = 0$ and $d_0^{(M)}(q) = d_0^{(B)}(q)$, i.e., the identification region for $\tilde{p}_0$ is the same under the basic assumption as under the stronger monotonicity assumption. For $\tilde{p}_1$ however, we see that while $d_1^{(M)}(q) = d_1^{(B)}(q)$, it must be that $c_1^{(M)}(q) >$

$c_1^{(B)}(q) = 0$. That is, we have to increase z_1 above zero in order to map $\tilde{p}_1$ far enough southeast of $\tilde{q}_1$ to hit $\mathbb{T}_1$. Again it is quite cumbersome to give algebraic expressions for the $\mathbb{Z}_M(q)$ boundaries, though these are available in the online code. As a comment on how these are computed, it is helpful to consider four different cases, according to (i) whether $\tilde{q}_1$ is southeast or northwest of $\tilde{q}_0$, and (ii) whether the connecting line passes above or below the point $(a, b) = (1/3, 1/3)$. The latter is useful in determining which edges of $\mathbb{T}_0$ and $\mathbb{T}_1$ are involved, for cases where the $\tilde{p}_i$ identification region shrinks under the monotonicity assumption relative to the basic assumption.

Computing the Limiting Posterior Distribution

With the form of the identification region in hand, determining the LPD is relatively straightforward. We presume that the prior distribution is specified to be of the form

$$\pi(\theta) \propto \pi(p_0)\pi(p_1)\pi(r_0)\pi(r_1)I_A(p_0, p_1), \tag{4.2}$$

where A is taken to be either $\mathbb{P}_B$ or $\mathbb{P}_M$, as desired. That is, we start with *a priori* independence between p_0, p_1, r_0, r_1, and perhaps standard distributional forms, such as Dirichlet for each p_i and Beta for each r_i. Then we truncate to enforce either the basic assumption or the monotonicity assumption, generically indicated via the $I_A()$ indicator in (4.2).

Straightforward calculus exercises give

$$\left| \frac{\partial \phi, \lambda}{\partial \theta} \right| = \frac{1}{|r_1 - r_0|}$$

and

$$\left| \frac{\partial \theta}{\partial \phi, \lambda} \right| = \frac{1}{|1 + z_0 + z_1|},$$

which, as a check on calculation, are easily verified to behave reciprocally. Hence the LPD is characterized by a point-mass distribution for $q = q^\dagger$ along with the bivariate distribution on $z = (z_0, z_1)$ having density proportional to $\pi(\theta(q^\dagger, z))|1 + z_0 + z_1|^{-1}I_A(p_0(q^\dagger, z_0), p_1(q^\dagger, z_1))$. We then have a recipe to evaluate the unnormalized density on a two-dimensional grid of z values. Alternately, a simple Monte Carlo strategy is to simulate realizations of z^* from the uniform distribution over the rectangular region $\mathbb{Z}_A(q)$. The requisite importance weights to make the realizations representative of the LPD must then take the form

$$w(z) \propto \frac{\pi(\theta(q^\dagger, z))\left(d_0^{(A)}(q^\dagger) - c_0^{(A)}(q^\dagger)\right)\left(d_1^{(A)}(q^\dagger) - c_1^{(A)}(q^\dagger)\right)}{|1 + z_0 + z_1|}. \tag{4.3}$$

Computing the Posterior Distribution

In fact this Monte Carlo scheme is easily adapted to perform finite-sample inference, as a version of the importance sampling strategy outlined in Section 2.3. As a convenience prior we could take

$$\pi^*(q,z) \quad \propto \quad I\{q \in \mathbb{Q}_A\} \times \frac{I\{z \in \mathbb{Z}_A(q)\}}{\|\mathbb{Z}_A(q)\|},$$

where $\| \bullet \|$ gives the area of a set in the plane. Less algebraically, under π^* marginally q is distributed such that q_0^* and q_1^* are independent Dirichlet$(1,1,1)$ realizations, but then truncated to ensure the connecting line is compatible with whichever assumption (basic or monotone) imposed. Then the conditional distribution of z given q is simply uniform over the identification region. Exact sampling from the convenience posterior is then trivial, as the q marginal involves $q_i^* \sim$ Dirichlet$(1+n_{i0}, 1+n_{i1}, 1+n_{i2})$, again truncated to $q^* \in \mathbb{Q}_A$. And the $(z|q)$ conditional posterior is the same as the conditional prior. The requisite importance sampling weights $w(q,z)$ simply take the same form as (4.3), but with $q^\dagger$ replaced by q.

Demonstration

Figure 4.2 gives examples of the bivariate posterior distribution on $r = (r_0, r_1)$ attained from both finite and infinite sample sizes. Throughout, the data "cell proportions" are fixed as $n_{0+}^{-1}(n_{00}, n_{01}, n_{02}) = (0.492, 0.108, 0.400)$ and $n_{1+}^{-1}(n_{10}, n_{11}, n_{12}) = (0.313, 0.087, 0.600)$. It is easy to check that these proportions correspond to points outside of $\mathbb{T}_0$ and $\mathbb{T}_1$, respectively, but the connecting line is compatible with the monotonicity assumption. Using the importance sampling strategy, the posterior marginal distributions are given when the sample sizes are (i) $n_{0+} = n_{1+} = 250$, (ii) $n_{0+} = n_{1+} = 1000$, and (iii) $n_{0+} = n_{1+} = \infty$. This is done for both the basic assumption and the monotonicity assumption.

Under the basic assumption, and with $n_{i+} = 250$, we see a posterior marginal that is somewhat informative relative to the prior marginal (whereby r is uniformly distributed over the unit square). And this posterior distribution is conclusive in establishing that $r_1 > r_0$. On the other hand, diminishing returns are at play, with very little further posterior concentration exhibited in moving to $n_{i+} = 1000$, or even $n_{i+} = \infty$. Under the monotonicity assumption, at each sample size we see a posterior on r that is considerably tightened relative to its counterpart under the basic assumption. Moreover, in this case there is considerable concentration of the posterior accruing from increasing sample size.

As a final illustration using these cell proportions, we take a look at the LPD for the log odds-ratio $\psi = \text{logit } r_1 - \text{logit } r_0$ in Figure 4.3. We have already

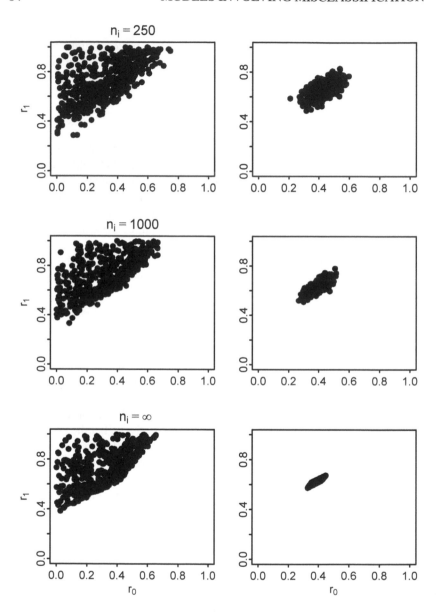

Figure 4.2 *Posterior distribution of prevalences* $r_y = Pr(X = 1|Y = y)$ *in Example D, for fixed cell proportions but increasing sample size. The left and right panels correspond to the basic assumption and the monotonicity assumption, respectively. In all cases the plots contain 500 points resampled from the importance sampling output of size* $30,000$ *according to the importance weights. Across the six analyses, the effective sample size ranges from 7,300 to 10,000.*

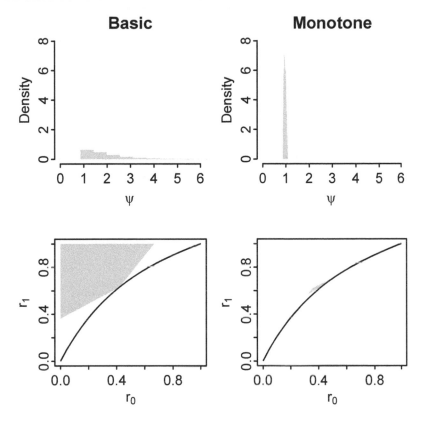

Figure 4.3 *Limiting posterior distribution on the log odds-ratio in Example D, under the basic and monotonicity assumptions (upper panels). The values of q are given in the text. The lower panels illustrate how both identification regions yield the same lower bound on the odds ratio, as attained at the common vertex of the two regions. The indicated curves are contours of constant odds-ratio.*

seen in Figure 4.2 that the identification region for (r_0, r_1) is far smaller under the monotonicity assumption than under the basic assumption. This translates to a much more concentrated LPD on ψ. In fact, though, the difference is all down to the right-tail of the LPD. Quite generally, the geometry of the identification region for r is such that the southeast vertex of the polygonal boundary is common under both assumptions. Moreover, the minimum odds ratio will occur at this vertex, given the shape of constant odds-ratio contours, as portrayed in the lower panels of Figure 4.3. Generally, these sorts of geometric insights are gathered together in Wang et al. (2012), as follows.

Presume that the $\tilde{q}$ connecting line is compatible with the basic constraint. Also, assume without loss of generality that $\tilde{q}_1$ is southeast of $\tilde{q}_0$ (as must arise if $r_1 > r_0$, so that a *lower bound* on the odds-ratio will be a bound away from the null). Then we have the following:

• Making only the basic assumption, the upper bound on the odds-ratio will be infinite.

• Provided $\tilde{q}$ is compatible with the monotonicity assumption, invoking the basic assumption or invoking the monotonicity assumption will yield the same lower bound on the odds-ratio.

• Provided $\tilde{q}$ is compatible with the monotonicity assumption, if $\tilde{q} \in \mathbb{P}_M$, then $\mathbb{Z}_B = \mathbb{Z}_M$, i.e., either assumption lead to the same identification region in such cases.

• Provided $\tilde{q}$ is compatible with the monotonicity assumption, a finite upper-bound on the odds-ratio obtains under this assumption if and only if $\tilde{q}_0$ lies outside $\mathbb{T}_0$ and $\tilde{q}_1$ lies outside $\mathbb{T}_1$.

In all, this example serves to illustrate several common features of partially identified models. First, the strength of background assumptions (here either the basic assumption or the monotonicity assumption) can have a strong influence on the identification region. Second, the amount of learning from data can vary widely with changes in the underlying parameter values. In particular, under the monotonicity assumption we might obtain a finite upper-bound on the odds-ratio, or we might not. ∎

4.2 Binary Misclassification across Three Populations

We now revert to the situation of a binary surrogate X^* for a binary variable X, as per Example C from Chapter 3. Recall this example involved X^* being observable in two distinct samples from two populations (the controls and the cases), and we made the nondifferential misclassification assumption, namely that given X, the surrogate X^* is conditionally independent of the case/control status indicator Y.

In fact there is a rich literature on many variants of this situation, with principal considerations being (i) the number of different observable surrogates available for X, (ii) the number of distinct populations that can be sampled, and (iii) if there are multiple surrogates, then what, if anything, can be assumed about the dependence between them. Some references include Qu et al. (1996); Hui and Zhou (1998); Goetghebeur et al. (2000); Pepe and Janes (2007). Note also that inferential goals can be varied. In some applications the properties of the surrogates (e.g., sensitivity and specificity) are of primary interest, with the distribution of X across populations relegated to a nuisance parameter role. In other settings though, and particularly in the case-control setting, how the distribution X varies with Y is of interest, while the properties of the surrogates are nuisance parameters.

The first intuitions about identification in such problems tend to arise from parameter counting arguments. For instance, say that X is unobservable but has two observable surrogates, X_1^* and X_2^*. Also, say that two distinct populations can be sampled, with the case-control setting being a primary example where this arises. Moreover, say the surrogates are thought to be blind to Y, in the sense that (X_1^*, X_2^*) can be assumed to be conditionally independent of Y given X. And, finally, say that the two surrogates are thought to operate in a fundamentally different manner, such that X_1^* and X_2^* are conditionally independent of one another given X. Under this framework, we can count two parameters needed to describe the distribution of $(X|Y)$, two parameters needed to describe $(X_1^*|X)$, and two parameters needed to describe $(X_2^*|X)$. With the given conditional independencies, this completely determines the $(X, X_1^*, X_2^*|Y)$ distribution, and hence the $(X_1^*, X_2^*|Y)$ distribution which is learnable from the observable data. We then have the possibility that the distribution of observables completely determines all six parameters, since inherently $(X_1^*, X_2^*|Y)$ is a 6 degree-of-freedom entity.

By itself, this counting argument does not *prove* identification. However, Hui and Walter (1980) give an explicit expression inverting the map from the initial six parameters to the six cell probabilities characterizing $(X_1^*, X_2^*|Y)$. This confirms the suspicion that the model is identified. Perhaps it can also be viewed as a triumph of mathematics over intuition, since the latter suggests it should not be possible to learn about how X relates to Y without any *overt* information about the quality of the two surrogates for X.

Aside: An Identified Model with a "Danger-Zone"

It is worth noting that the inversion of Hui and Walter (1980) breaks down in the special case that X and Y are independent of one another. That is, as $Pr(X = 1|Y = 0)$ and $Pr(X = 1|Y = 1)$ tend toward one another, we transition from an identified situation to a nonidentified situation. In practice then it may be hard to estimate quantities if, in fact, $Pr(X = 1|Y = 1)$ is close to $Pr(X = 1|Y = 0)$. Gustafson (2005a,b) emphasizes this as an example of how identification issues can be nuanced, i.e., within an identified model parameter space there can be a lower-dimensional "danger-zone" of parameter values for which the distribution of the observables does not completely determine all the parameter values. In fact, in the present set-up this can be viewed as a "no free lunch" situation, and we should not be surprised that identification breaks down as the distribution of (X,Y) approaches independence. Were it otherwise, we could identify all the parameters in a one-population setting by using a randomized binary Y to fictitiously create two populations. But this just cannot happen, since the one-population version of the problem involves five unknown parameters but only three degrees of freedom for the (X_1^*, X_2^*) distribution of observables. So, the danger-zone within the identified model can actually be regarded as a feature, not a bug.★

Formally, the assumption of *nondifferential* surrogates, whereby (X_1^*, X_2^*) are conditionally independent of the population indicator Y given the true X, may be reasonable for some applications. For instance, an obvious "fit" with this mathematical story arises if a human rater determining a surrogate is indeed blinded to the Y values of the subjects rated. On the other hand, the assumption of conditional independence *between* two surrogates given the true X is often much harder to justify. It is easy to imagine that often X_1^* and X_2^* could be positively dependent given X, for one or both of $X = 0$ and $X = 1$. This could arise if some subjects are generally harder to correctly classify than others, across both techniques. Hence there is interest in relaxing this assumption. Clearly this is problematic in the two-population setting, as the $(X_1^*, X_2^*|Y)$ data still only provide six degrees of freedom, while eight unknown parameters are now at play: two describing $(X|Y)$ and three each describing $(X_1^*, X_2^*|X = x)$, for $x = 0$ and $x = 1$. However, the parameter counting argument becomes favorable in the face of more than two populations. In light of this, we turn our attention to the three-population scenario.

Example E: Misclassification across Three Populations

Let membership in one of three disjoint populations be indicated by $Y = 0$, $Y = 1$, and $Y = 2$, respectively. Retaining the nondifferential assumption that (X_1^*, X_2^*) are conditionally independent of Y given X, parameter counting does indeed suggest hope of identification. The $(X_1^*, X_2^*|Y)$ conditional distribution could support the estimation of up to nine parameters. And indeed nine parameters are at play: three describing $(X|Y)$ and three each describing $(X_1^*, X_2^*|X = x)$, for $x = 0$ and $x = 1$. However, this example illustrates that the number of unknown parameters being less than or equal to the data degrees-of-freedom is only a necessary condition for identification. It is not sufficient. In fact, Hanson and Johnson (2005) prove that the nine parameters are *not* completely determined by the nine cell probabilities characterizing $(X_1^*, X_2^*|Y)$. So, the parameter count notwithstanding, we are still squarely in the realm of partial identification.

Transparent Reparameterization

On first glance it is not obvious how to construct a transparent parameterization for this problem. Since three bivariate binary distributions are characterized by nine cell probabilities, it would seem that $\dim(\phi) = 9$ would be required. However, this would imply $\dim(\lambda) = \dim(\theta) - \dim(\phi) = 0$, which is nonsensical. This issue prompted Gustafson (2009) to attack the problem with a more complicated technique not requiring a transparent parameterization. It turns out though that the problem can be cast into our simpler framework, as we shall describe.

Let the initial parameterization for our problem be the nine parameters

$$\theta = (r_0, r_1, r_2, p_{000}, p_{010}, p_{001}, p_{100}, p_{110}, p_{101}),$$

where

$$r_y = Pr(X = 1 | Y = y),$$

and

$$p_{xab} = Pr(X_1^* = a, X_2^* = b | X = x),$$

noting that $p_{x11} = 1 - p_{x00} - p_{x10} - p_{x01}$ is implicitly defined. To give a transparent parameterization with $\dim(\lambda) = 2$, we take the seven components of ϕ to be

$$\phi = (q_{000}, q_{010}, q_{001}, q_{100}, q_{110}, q_{101}, \varepsilon). \tag{4.4}$$

Here,

$$\begin{aligned} q_{yab} &= Pr(X_1^* = a, X_2^* = b | Y = y) \\ &= (1 - r_y)p_{0ab} + r_y p_{1ab}, \end{aligned}$$

and

$$\varepsilon = (r_2 - r_1)/(r_1 - r_0).$$

Initially ϕ appears to have too few components. The distribution of $(X_1^*, X_2^* | Y = y)$ is characterized by $q_y = (q_{y00}, q_{y10}, q_{y01})$, so the omission of $q_{2\bullet\bullet}$ from (4.4) would seem to violate the requirement that ϕ determine the distribution of the observable data. However,

$$\begin{aligned} q_{2ab} &= (1 - r_2)p_{0ab} + r_2 p_{1ab} \\ &= [1 - \{r_1 + \varepsilon(r_2 - r_1)\}]p_{0ab} + \{r_1 + \varepsilon(r_2 - r_1)\}p_{1ab} \\ &= q_{1ab} + \varepsilon(q_{1ab} - q_{0ab}), \end{aligned}$$

evincing that ϕ does indeed completely describe the distribution of the observable data, while not being any bigger than necessary to fulfill this role. This clears up some of the confusion concerning the parameter counting issue. Presuming that the model assumptions are correct, we see that the data inherently possess only 7 degrees of freedom. Geometrically this can be viewed in terms of the three vectors of (X_1^*, X_2^*) cell probabilities for the three populations being collinear in the space of possible cell probabilities. Hence given two of the three vectors, the value of the third vector is described by a scalar reflecting its location along the line passing through the other two.

The transparent parameterization is completed by selecting two functions of θ to play the role of λ. A convenient choice is $\lambda = (\lambda_0, \lambda_1) = (r_0, r_1)$. The map from θ to (ϕ, λ) can then be inverted explicitly as

$$
\begin{aligned}
p_{0\bullet\bullet} &= (\lambda_0 - \lambda_1)^{-1}(\lambda_0 q_{1\bullet} - \lambda_1 q_{0\bullet}) \\
p_{1\bullet\bullet} &= (\lambda_1 - \lambda_0)^{-1}\{(1 - \lambda_0)q_{1\bullet\bullet} - (1 - \lambda_1)q_{0\bullet\bullet}\} \\
r_0 &= \lambda_0 \\
r_1 &= \lambda_1 \\
r_2 &= \lambda_1 + \varepsilon(\lambda_1 - \lambda_0).
\end{aligned}
\tag{4.5}
$$

Also, for future reference, direct calculation gives

$$
\left| \frac{\partial(\phi, \lambda)}{\partial \theta} \right| = (r_1 - r_0)^2,
$$

and commensurately

$$
\left| \frac{\partial \theta}{\partial(\phi, \lambda)} \right| = (\lambda_1 - \lambda_0)^{-2}.
$$

Determining the Identification Region

We now start to see some similarities with Example D from earlier in this chapter. Just as there, we have p describing the distribution of $(X^*|X)$ and r describing the distribution of $(X|Y)$, leading to q describing the observable distribution of $(X^*|Y)$. We are now much harder pressed to visualize the situation, since $p_{x\bullet\bullet}$ and $q_{y\bullet\bullet}$ have three free components rather than two. But the logic of determining the identification region remains the same. For given $\phi^\dagger = (q_{0\bullet\bullet}^\dagger, q_{1\bullet\bullet}^\dagger, \varepsilon^\dagger)$, and absent further assumptions, the identification region can be expressed as all values of $\lambda \in (0,1)^2$ for which the inverse mapping (4.5) yields a legitimate value in the original parameter space, i.e., $\theta \in \Theta$.

To give a specific example, say that the true characteristics of the two surrogates are $SP_1 = Pr(X_1^* = 0|X = 0) = 0.85$, $SP_2 = Pr(X_2^* = 0|X = 0) = 0.7$, $OR_0 = OR(X_1^*, X_2^*|X = 0) = 1.5$, $SN_1 = Pr(X_1^* = 1|X = 1) = 0.73$, $SN_2 =$

$Pr(X_2^* = 1 | X = 1) = 0.9$, $OR_1 = OR(X_1^*, X_2^* | X = 1) = 1.7$. This defines $p_{0\bullet\bullet}^{\dagger}$ and $p_{1\bullet\bullet}^{\dagger}$, though a little work is required in this step. For instance, the specificity values immediately give the margins as $p_{000} + p_{001} = SP_1$ and $p_{000} + p_{010} = SP_2$. Then OR_0 completes the specification, with the proviso that it is necessary to solve a quadratic equation, i.e., solve

$$OR_0 = \frac{p_{000}(1 + p_{000} - SP_1 - SP_2)}{(SP_1 - p_{000})(SP_2 - p_{000})}$$

for p_{000}. An analogous argument also yields the elements of $p_{1\bullet\bullet}$ given (SN_1, SN_2, OR_1). Also for our example, we set $(r_0^{\dagger}, r_1^{\dagger}, r_2^{\dagger}) = (0.15, 0.4, 0.7)$, such that the exposure prevalence varies dramatically across the three populations.

For this setting of $(\phi^{\dagger}, \lambda^{\dagger}) = h(\theta^{\dagger})$ we depict the identification region in Figure 4.4. For each point on a two-dimensional grid of $(\lambda_0, \lambda_1) = (r_0, r_1)$ values, we simply test for inclusion in the identification region by checking whether $h^{-1}(\phi^{\dagger}, \lambda)$ as given above lies in the parameter space. This identification region is illustrated in the upper-left panel of the figure. Presuming all three exposure prevalences are of interest, however, we also present the region in terms of (r_1, r_2) and in terms of (r_0, r_2). This works in that given $\phi^{\dagger}$, any two of the prevalences uniquely determine the third.

From the plots it is clear that without further assumptions we have a serious issue. The identification region is composed of two disjoint sets, with one obtained via 180 degree rotation of the other. Or, more algebraically, $(r_0, r_1) = (a, b)$ is in the identification region if and only if $(r_0, r_1) = (1 - a, 1 - b)$ is in the region. Put roughly then, without further assumptions we learn something from the data, but we do not know if we are learning the prevalences of $X = 1$ or the prevalences of $X = 0$. In the figure we have the luxury of knowing all the true parameter values, consequently we know which of the two subsets contains the true values. Of course real applications are not accompanied by such luxuries.

This situation can be resolved if, as with related examples, we assume that the surrogates are better than random. Assuming $SN_1 + SP_1 > 1$ and $SN_2 + SP_2 > 1$ corresponds to further requiring that $(\phi^{\dagger}, \lambda)$ gets mapped to a value of θ with $p_{110} + p_{111} + p_{000} + p_{001} > 1$ and $p_{101} + p_{111} + p_{000} + p_{010} > 1$. This indeed resolves the "which level of X is which" conundrum, by removing the wrong subset from the identification region.

Another plausible assumption in many applications would be that any dependence between X_1^* and X_2^* must be positive, corresponding to $p_{x11}p_{x00} \geq p_{x10}p_{x01}$ for $x = 0, 1$. We see in Figure 4.4 that adding this assumption yields a further modest reduction in the size of the identification region. Generally, note that the two assumptions produce an identification region that, when expressed in terms of any pair of prevalences, lies well to one side of the identity line.

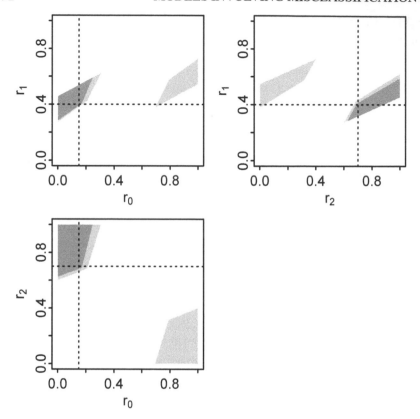

Figure 4.4 *Identification region for (r_0, r_1, r_2) in Example E, when the true parameter values are $(r_0, r_1, r_2) = (0.15, 0.4, 0.7)$, $(SP_1, SP_2, OR_0) = (0.85, 0.7, 1.5)$, $(SN_1, SN_2, OR_1) = (0.73, 0.9, 1.7)$. The union of the light-grey and dark-grey regions corresponds to the identification region without extra assumptions. The dark-grey region alone is the identification region after further assuming that (i) both surrogates for X are better than random, and (ii) ruling out negative dependence between the two surrogates given true exposure. For reference, the dotted lines indicate the true values.*

Thus, the lack of full identification notwithstanding, data can unequivocally order the three populations for us, from lowest to highest X prevalence.

As alluded to previously, an inconvenient truth about partially identified models is that estimator performance can vary dramatically with the true values of the underlying parameters. Consider, for instance, keeping $p_{0\bullet\bullet}^{\dagger}$ and $p_{1\bullet\bullet}^{\dagger}$ as above, but changing the exposure prevalences to be much less separated. Particularly, we take $(r_0^{\dagger}, r_1^{\dagger}, r_2^{\dagger}) = (0.1, 0.2, 0.3)$. The corresponding identification region, given in Figure 4.5, is far larger than in the previous setting. Nonetheless, note that for each pair of prevalences the region lies wholly on one side

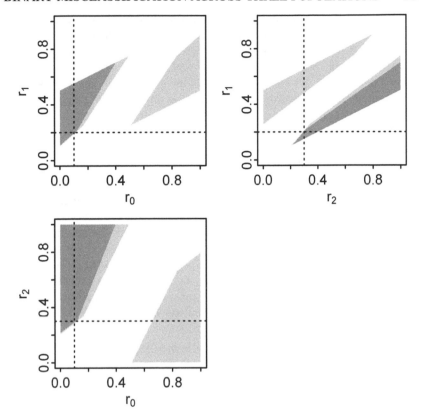

Figure 4.5 *Identification region for* (r_0, r_1, r_2) *in Example E, when the true pa-rameter values are* $(r_0, r_1, r_2) = (0.1, 0.2, 0.3)$, $(SP_1, SP_2, OR_0) = (0.85, 0.7, 1.5)$, $(SN_1, SN_2, OR_1) = (0.73, 0.9, 1.7)$. *The format is as per Figure 4.4.*

of the identity line. So, while there is less information about each prevalence in this setting, with enough data one would still learn their order correctly.

Determining the Limiting Posterior Distribution

We now move on to consider the limiting posterior distribution for this exam-ple. We presume a uniform prior distribution in the initial parameterization, appropriately truncated. More formally, we start with $r_i^\star \sim \mathrm{Uniform}(0, 1)$ for $i = 0, 1, 2$, and $p_{x\bullet\bullet}^\star \sim \mathrm{Dirichlet}(1, 1, 1, 1)$ for $x = 0, 1$, all mutually indepen-dent. Then, however, the constant density function is truncated to only those values for which both surrogates are better than random, and the conditional dependence between surrogates is non-negative.

Our scheme for determining whether a given value of λ is in the identification region for a given value of ϕ is algorithmic, rather than algebraically characterized. Consequently, we lack an efficient choice of convenience prior $\pi^*(\lambda|\phi)$, and simply make do with the inefficient choice of a bivariate uniform distribution on $(0,1)^2$. We know that many of the generated points will accrue zero weight as they fall outside the identification region, but the algorithm is still valid. In light of the Jacobian term given earlier, we know that the weight for a generated value of $\lambda = (r_0, r_1)$ will simply be

$$w(r_0, r_1) \quad = \quad \frac{I_{A(\phi)}(r_0, r_1)}{(r_1 - r_0)^2}. \tag{4.6}$$

For the first setting of $\phi^\dagger$ above, the marginal distributions of the limiting posterior appear in Figure 4.6. We see that the shape of each posterior marginal distribution across the corresponding "margin" of the identification region is not uniform, despite the uniform prior specification. Against this, however, most of the limiting posterior marginals are somewhat close to flat in shape, with those for r_1, LOR_0 and LOR_1 being the notable exceptions. In practical terms, LOR_0 and LOR_1 retain the most uncertainty *a priori*, giving considerable weight to very strong conditional association for $(X_1^*, X_2^*|X)$, but not ruling out a complete lack of association.

Turning to the second set of $\phi^\dagger$ values, as arises from much less discrepant prevalences $(r_0^\dagger, r_1^\dagger r_2^\dagger) = (0.1, 0.2, 0.3)$, the resulting limiting posterior marginal densities appear in Figure 4.7. The theme that estimator performance can vary dramatically across underlying parameter values in partially identified contexts is reinforced here. Compared to the first setting, we see less information about $(r_0, r_1, r_2, SN_1, SN_2)$, but more information about (SP_1, SP_2). To some extent this is intuitive, in that the present setting corresponds to lower X prevalences, hence more opportunity to learn about specificity and less to learn about sensitivity. Again in this setting, the information about the conditional association between the surrogates X_1^* and X_2^* given X is quite weak.

Alternative Prior Distributions

As always with partially identified models, a lurking question is to what extent does the choice of prior distribution drive the posterior distribution, even in the large-sample limit. We have already made note of the wide limiting posterior distributions on the association parameters. Additionally, we note that the shape of these limiting posterior distributions favors very strong associations over a lack of association, whereas in practice an assumption that the dependence is unlikely to be very strong might be warranted. Thus we investigate what happens when we change the prior accordingly.

To specify a prior which puts more weight on weaker associations, we follow Gustafson (2009). For instance, consider $p_{0\bullet\bullet}$ describing the distribution

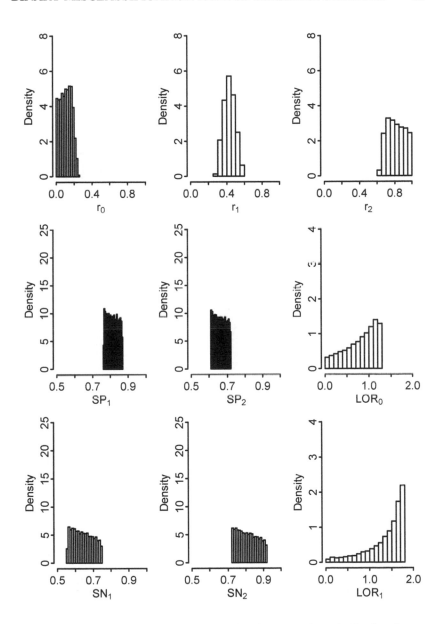

Figure 4.6 *Margins of the limiting posterior distribution in Example E, when the true parameter values are* $(r_0, r_1, r_2) = (0.15, 0.4, 0.7)$, $(SP_1, SP_2, OR_0) = (0.85, 0.7, 1.5)$, $(SN_1, SN_2, OR_1) = (0.73, 0.9, 1.7)$. *These were computed from a Monte Carlo sample of size* 10^6, *resulting in* $33,300$ *points with positive weight, and an effective sample size of* $29,900$. *Note that* $LOR_x = \log OR(X_1^*, X_2^* | X = x)$.

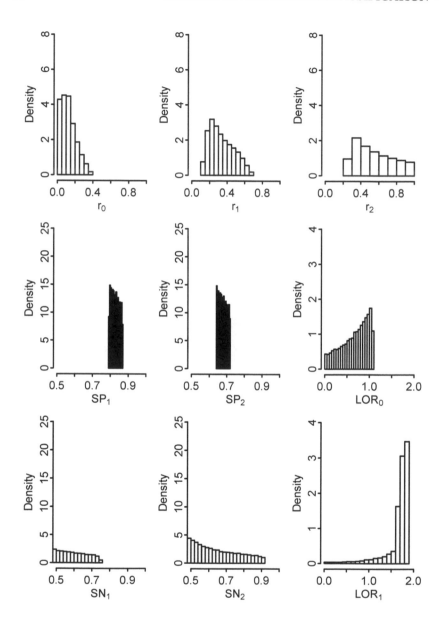

Figure 4.7 *Margins of the limiting posterior distribution in Example E, when the true parameter values are* $(r_0, r_1, r_2) = (0.1, 0.2, 0.3)$, $(SP_1, SP_2, OR_0) = (0.85, 0.7, 1.5)$, $(SN_1, SN_2, OR_1) = (0.73, 0.9, 1.7)$. *These were computed from a Monte Carlo sample of size* 10^6, *resulting in* 92,800 *points with positive weight, and an effective sample size of* 50,800. *Note that* $LOR_x = \log OR(X_1^*, X_2^* | X = x)$.

of $(X_1^*, X_2^* | X = 0)$. We could start with a distribution under which SP_1, SP_2 and $\log OR(X_1^*, X_2^* | X = 0)$ are independent, with standard uniform marginals in the first two instances, and an exponential distribution with mean m in the latter case. We can take the same prior structure for $p_{1\bullet\bullet}$ describing $(X_1^*, X_2^* | X = 1)$, and retain uniform prior distributions on each r_i. Transforming this distribution to our parameterization, and truncating such that the surrogates are better than random and the associations are non-negative, we have

$$\pi(\theta) \quad \propto \quad I_A(\theta) \prod_{x=0}^{1} \exp\{-s(p_{x\bullet\bullet})/m\} \left(\frac{1}{p_{x00}} + \frac{1}{p_{x01}} + \frac{1}{p_{x10}} + \frac{1}{p_{x11}} \right),$$

where $s(p_{x\bullet\bullet}) = \log p_{x00} + \log p_{x11} - \log p_{x01} - \log p_{x10}$ is the log odds-ratio for $(X_1^*, X_2^* | X = x)$, while the set A restricts to us to better-than-random surrogates with nonnegative dependence.

In turn, we can go after the LPD using importance sampling, again using bivariate uniform draws. Rather than (4.6), we now get importance weights of the form

$$w(r_0, r_1) \quad = \quad \frac{I_{A(\phi^\dagger)}(r_0, r_1) \pi(\theta(\phi^\dagger, r_0, r_1))}{(r_1 - r_0)^2}.$$

This computational scheme is even less efficient than before, but still can be made to work. The limiting posterior marginals under this choice of prior with $m = \log 2$ appear in Figure 4.8 for the first parameter setting and in Figure 4.9 for the second setting. The results confirm that the limiting posterior marginals for the association parameter are very sensitive to the prior specifications for these parameters. One can see that moving to a prior favoring weaker associations indeed pushes the posterior in the commensurate direction. But beyond that, the mild infusion of prior information on the association parameters leads to considerable sharpening of the marginal posteriors on the "main" parameters, i.e, (r_0, r_1, r_2), (SP_1, SP_2), and (SN_1, SN_2). This would seem to involve "good bang for the buck." If it is defensible to assert a priori that very strong conditional associations between surrogates are unlikely, then demonstrably one can learn more about the other parameters. Again, this should really come as no surprise. Compared to the first prior specification, the second specification is downweighting larger departures from the identified model involving conditionally independent surrogates.

Finite-Sample Demonstration

Finally with this example, we turn our attention to finite-sample inference. Our first thought is to apply the importance sampling strategy outlined in Chapter 2. This requires a convenience marginal prior $\pi^*(\phi)$ for which Monte Carlo simulation from the corresponding posterior $\pi^*(\phi | d)$ is quite easy. In this problem,

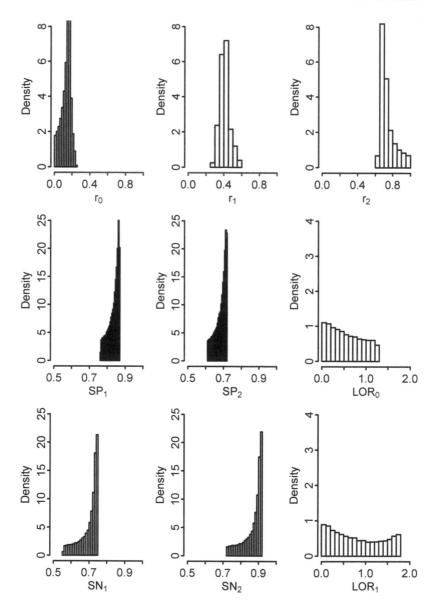

Figure 4.8 *Margins of the limiting posterior distribution in Example E, under the alternate prior distribution. The true parameter values are* $(r_0, r_1, r_2) = (0.15, 0.4, 0.7)$, $(SP_1, SP_2, OR_0) = (0.85, 0.7, 1.5)$, $(SN_1, SN_2, OR_1) = (0.73, 0.9, 1.7)$. *These were computed from a Monte Carlo sample of size* 5×10^6, *resulting in* 160,400 *points with positive weight, and an effective sample size of* 19,100. *Note that* $LOR_x = \log OR(X_1^*, X_2^* | X = x)$.

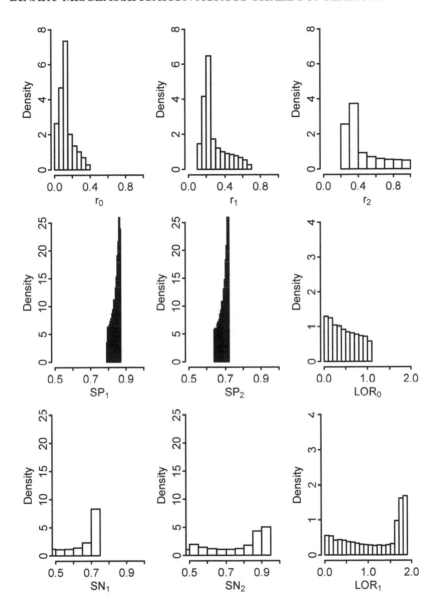

Figure 4.9 *Margins of the limiting posterior distribution in Example E, under the alternate prior distribution. The true parameter values are* $(r_0, r_1, r_2) = (0.1, 0.2, 0.3)$, $(SP_1, SP_2, OR_0) - (0.85, 0.7, 1.5)$, $(SN_1, SN_2, OR_1) - (0.73, 0.9, 1.7)$. *These were computed from a Monte Carlo sample of size* 5×10^6, *resulting in* 463,600 *points with positive weight, and an effective sample size of* 13,900. *Note that* $LOR_x = \log OR(X_1^*, X_2^* | X = x)$.

however, we are rather stymied on how to make this work. While we could set up a conjugate prior for $q_{0\bullet\bullet}$ and $q_{1\bullet\bullet}$ for updating with the data from the first two populations only, our conjugate structure is destroyed upon trying to incorporate the remaining parameter ε and the data from the third population.

We could attempt to use MCMC to simulate from $\pi(\phi|d)$, but if we have to go to the bother of using MCMC, we may as well apply it to the whole posterior distribution. In fact, we can simply adopt the MCMC algorithm proposed in Gustafson (2009) for this model. Briefly, this algorithm operates via random-walk Metropolis-Hastings updates (Hastings, 1970; Tierney, 1994) applied to three blocks of parameters: (r_0, r_1, r_2), $(SP_1, SP_2, \log OR_0)$, and $(SN_1, SN_2, \log OR_1)$. As is customary with this algorithm, it is "fiddly" in that the jump size for each of the three updates must be tuned in order to obtain a mid-range acceptance probability. And, as always with MCMC, one must look at the output with an eye to convergence and mixing behavior.

As a brief demonstration of the evolution of finite-sample inference, we simulate a telescoping data sequence using our first setting for the underlying parameters (with the spread out X prevalences particularly), and the prior which mildly penalizes strong conditional association between the surrogates. That is, we are precisely in the setting of Figure 4.8. Using the notation n_{yab} as the number of subjects with $(Y = y, X_1^* = a, X_2^* = b)$, we take equal-sized samples from each population, i.e, $n_{y++} = n$, for $y = 0, 1, 2$, with "stops" at $n = 100$, $n = 400$, and $n = 1600$. In Figure 4.10 we give tri-interval plots for the posterior marginal distributions of both r_1 and SN_2, with the LPDs as per Figure 4.8 also included.

Again, the results fit the partially identified model mould. The first $n = 100$ observations (per population) give good accumulation of knowledge relative to the diffuse prior distributions for these two parameters. Then the first quadrupling of sample size is quite effective in further reducing uncertainty, though not quite by the factor of two seen in identified settings. Subsequently, diminishing returns set in, with scant further posterior concentration as data accumulate. Having said that, though, the case of SN_2 deserves special comment. Here the LPD is very highly skewed, with density increasing dramatically over the identification interval (this is clearest in Figure 4.9). What we see in going from $n = 400$ to $n = 1600$ to $n = \infty$ is little change in the 95% HPD interval, but marked concentration and increase in the 50% HPD interval. Roughly put, the posterior finds the right support quite quickly as the data accrue, but the highly skewed shape emerges later in the data evolution. ∎

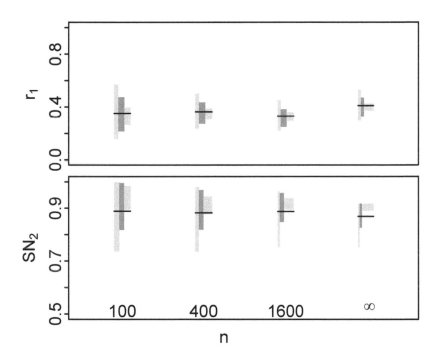

Figure 4.10 *Finite-sample evolution of the posterior marginal distributions of r_1 and SN_2 in Example E, with n observations from each of the three populations. The underlying parameter values and choice of prior distribution are as per Figure 4.8. For finite n, the posterior is determined via 100,000 MCMC iterations obtained after 5,000 burn-in iterations.*

Chapter 5

Further Examples: Models Involving Instrumental Variables

5.1 What is an Instrumental Variable?

Our starting point for discussing instrumental variables is that we would like to be able to regress an outcome variable Y on explanatory variables X and U, with particular interest in the role of X in the conditional distribution of $(Y|X,U)$. That is, we would like to infer the X-Y association *adjusted* for U, and we might refer to U as a *confounder*, or at least a *potential confounder*. A serious challenge arises, however, in that while X and Y are observable, U is unobservable. The hope is that a different observable variable Z, having special properties, can save the day.

With respect to (Y,X,U), Z is an *instrumental variable* (IV) if:

(i) Z is associated with X;

(ii) Z is independent of U;

(iii) Z is conditionally independent of Y given (X,U).

Roughly put, the force of these assumptions is to say that Z can only influence Y via X. Consequently, the magnitude of the observable association between Z and Y carries information about the influence of X on Y conditioned on U.

While this simple framework for an instrumental variable suffices for the purposes of this chapter, many applications involve the desire to adjust for the unobservable confounder U in addition to some observable confounders $C = (C_1, \ldots, C_m)$. In this case the assumptions generalize naturally to conditional association of $(Z,X|C)$, conditional independence of $(Z,U|C)$, and conditional independence of $(Z,Y|U,C)$. While instrumental variable methods have very longstanding roots in the econometrics literature and economic applications, in recent times they have gained some traction in the biostatistical and epidemiological spheres. For some relatively recent introductions from this perspective, see Newhouse and McClellan (1998), Greenland (2000), Hernán and Robins (2006), and Rassen et al. (2009).

When viewed mathematically as a set of three assumptions, the IV framework can look a little arbitrary. To add some intuition, consider the following "stock" example. If a study involves randomization to two or more treatment groups, then we hope for freedom from worry about confounding variables. The randomization will approximately balance these variables across treatment groups. However, this hope can be dampened in contexts where study subjects may not comply with their randomized assignment. Think of Z as indicating the treatment to which a subject is randomly assigned. For concreteness, we focus on the two-group case, where $Z = 0$ is assignment to the control or placebo group, and $Z = 1$ is assignment to the "active-treatment" group. In contrast, let X indicate treatment actually received, again either control or active treatment. Thus noncompliance arises if $X \neq Z$ for some subjects. And the worry with noncompliance is that an unobservable variable U might influence both the choice to comply and the outcome Y. This creates a desire to adjust for U, despite it being unobserved. We are on firm ground with the IV assumptions here, since the randomization will influence X as per (i), but is inherently unable to influence U, or to influence to the outcome other than via X. So (ii) and (iii) are justified.

It is not so surprising that identification issues arise with instrumental variable models, given that trying to adjust for U without observing U is pushing up against the boundaries of what is statistically possible. In this chapter we first study a variant of the IV problem which is only partially identified even with the IV assumptions invoked. And then we consider a problem where partial identification arises from weakening the assumptions.

5.2 Imperfect Compliance

Example F: Imperfect Compliance in a Randomized Trial

Here we pursue the setting mentioned above, of a randomized trial with imperfect compliance to treatment assignment. The two-treatment situation is assumed, so that binary Z and X indicate assigned and actual treatment status, respectively. Colloquially, we will refer to "not taking" and "taking" treatment, as per a study with a control group and an active-treatment group. The outcome Y is also presumed to be binary. To reflect the possibility of confounding between compliance behavior and outcome, we simply take U to be the trinary variable indicating whether a subject is someone who will comply with their assignment no matter what, someone who will choose to remain untreated no matter what, or someone who will choose to be treated no matter what. Rather than writing $U \in \{0,1,2\}$ to denote these three levels, it is more evocative to write $U \in \{c,n,a\}$, to indicate compliers, never-takers, and always-takers, respectively. This approach to the compliance issue in randomized studies has been studied by several authors, including Chickering and Pearl (1996), Imbens and Rubin (1997), and Pearl (2000), and has come to be known as one application of *principal stratification*, as codified by Frangakis and Rubin (2002). It should be mentioned that the trinary categorization of U rules out the possibility that anyone is a defier, i.e., we assume nobody in the population is *a priori* guaranteed to disobey their assignment no matter which way it turns out. However, more general treatments of the problem do allow for defiers (Richardson et al., 2011).

Parameterizations

With (Z,X,Y,U) defined as above, and invoking the IV assumptions, an initial parameterization of this problem is

$$\theta = (r_n, r_a, p_{c0}, p_{c1}, p_{n0}, p_{n1}, p_{a0}, p_{a1})$$

where $r_u = Pr(U = u)$, and $p_{ux} = Pr(Y = 1 | X = x, U = u)$. Note that $r_c = 1 - r_n - r_a$ is defined implicitly. Note also that some of the parameters have scientific meaning but no empirical meaning. For instance, $p_{n1} = Pr(Y = 1 | X = 1, U = n) = E(Y | X = 1, U = n)$ is the average response amongst never-takers who take treatment. Scientifically this is okay, as it is legitimate to think about how well never-takers would do if they were forced to take treatment. Of course empirically we will never see data on people with $(X = 1, U = n)$, and this contributes to the lack of identification. Nonetheless, we can still target a quantity such as

$$\psi = E\{E(Y | X = 1, U) - E(Y | X = 0, U)\}$$
$$= \sum_{u \in \{c,n,a\}} r_u(p_{u1} - p_{u0}) \tag{5.1}$$

for inference. This *average causal effect* (ACE) focuses on the effect of X within each stratum of U, averaged with respect to the proportion of the population in each stratum.

A transparent parameterization for this problem is based on

$$\phi = (q_{001}, q_{010}, q_{011}, q_{101}, q_{110}, q_{111}),$$

where

$$q_{zxy} = Pr(X = x, Y = y | Z = z)$$
$$= \sum_{u \in \{c,n,a\}} Pr(X = x, Y = y, U = u | Z = z)$$

$$
\begin{aligned}
= \ & \sum_{u \in \{c,n,a\}} Pr(Y=y|X=x,U=u,Z=z)Pr(X=x|U=u,Z=z) \ \times \\
& Pr(U=u|Z=z) \\
= \ & \sum_{u \in \{c,n,a\}} Pr(Y=y|X=x,U=u)Pr(X=x|U=u,Z=z)Pr(U=u) \\
= \ & \sum_{u \in \{c,n,a\}} p_{ux}^{y}(1-p_{ux})^{1-y}Pr(X=x|U=u,Z=z)r_u.
\end{aligned}
$$

Note here that in going from the third to fourth equalities both IV assumption (ii) and IV assumption (iii) are invoked. Note as well that $Pr(X=x|U=u,Z=z)$ is completely known, i.e., free of parameters. That is,

$$
Pr(X=1|U=u,Z=z) \quad = \quad
\begin{cases}
z & \text{if } u=c; \\
0 & \text{if } u=n; \\
1 & \text{if } u=a.
\end{cases}
$$

Also note that $q_{z00}=1-q_{z01}-q_{q10}-q_{z11}$ is implicitly defined, for $z=0,1$. And, finally, note that indeed the distribution of the observed data depends on θ only through ϕ. We can regard the data from those randomly assigned to control as a multinomial realization from $(Y,X|Z=0)$, as described by $q_{0\bullet\bullet}$. Similarly the data from those randomly assigned to treatment are viewed as a multinomial realization from $(Y,X|Z=1)$, as described by $q_{1\bullet\bullet}$.

Putting the pieces together, the mapping from θ to ϕ is more explicitly written as

$$
\begin{aligned}
q_{001} &= r_c p_{c0} + r_n p_{n0} \\
q_{010} &= r_a(1-p_{a1}) \\
q_{011} &= r_a p_{a1} \\
q_{111} &= r_c p_{c1} + r_a p_{a1} \\
q_{100} &= r_n(1-p_{n0}) \\
q_{101} &= r_n p_{n0}.
\end{aligned}
$$

Hence ϕ depends on only six of the eight components of θ, with p_{n1} and p_{a0} being the components that do not appear. This is intuitively sensible, in that the data do not contribute any information about the expected outcome for never-takers were they to take treatment, or the expected outcome for always-takers were they to not take treatment. Also, for future reference note that the Jacobian for the map from the six elements of θ to ϕ is given by

$$
\left| \frac{\partial q}{\partial (r_n \ r_a \ p_{c0} \ p_{c1} \ p_{n0} \ p_{a1})} \right| \quad = \quad (1-r_n-r_a)^2 r_n r_a. \tag{5.2}
$$

Computing the Limiting Posterior Distribution

In fact, the map from the six components of θ to q is readily seen to be invertible, by taking, in order,

$$
\begin{aligned}
p_{a1} &= \operatorname{expit}(\log q_{011} - \log q_{010}) \\
r_a &= q_{011}/p_{a1} \\
p_{n0} &= \operatorname{expit}(\log q_{101} - \log q_{100}) \\
r_n &= q_{101}/p_{n0} \\
p_{c0} &= (q_{001} - r_n p_{n0})/r_c \\
p_{c1} &= (q_{111} - r_a p_{a1})/r_c.
\end{aligned}
$$

So immediately we have the limiting posterior distribution characterized by a point-mass distribution on $(r_n, r_a, p_{c0}, p_{c1}, p_{n0}, p_{a1})$, along with the prior conditional distribution of $(p_{n1}, p_{a0} \mid r_n, r_a, p_{c0}, p_{c1}, p_{n0}, p_{a1})$.

Returning back to our inferential target, we thus have the marginal limiting posterior on the average causal effect ψ characterized stochastically as the distribution of

$$
\begin{aligned}
\psi^{\star} &= \left(1 - r_n^{\dagger} - r_c^{\dagger}\right)\left(p_{c1}^{\dagger} - p_{c0}^{\dagger}\right) + r_n^{\dagger}\left(p_{n1}^{\star} - p_{n0}^{\dagger}\right) + \\
&\quad r_a^{\dagger}\left(p_{a1}^{\dagger} - p_{a0}^{\star}\right),
\end{aligned}
\tag{5.3}
$$

as induced by the conditional prior density $\pi(p_{n1}, p_{a0} \mid r_n^{\dagger}, r_a^{\dagger}, p_{c0}^{\star}, p_{c1}^{\dagger}, p_{n0}^{\dagger}, p_{a1}^{\dagger})$. Presuming this conditional prior density is fully supported on $(0,1)^2$, the limiting posterior distribution for ψ is immediately seen to be supported on the identification region $a(\phi^{\dagger}) \pm b(\phi^{\dagger})$, where

$$
a(\phi) = (1 - r_n - r_c)(p_{c1} - p_{c0}) + r_n(1/2 - p_{n0}) + r_a(p_{a1} - 1/2),
$$

and

$$
b(\phi) = (r_n + r_a)/2.
$$

Note then that while we do learn the proportions of each compliance type in the population, we only learn the target completely if in fact there are only compliers in the population. And, as makes intuitive sense, a higher proportion of non-compliers goes hand in hand with less information about the target.

An interesting special case arises when (p_{n1}, p_{a0}) are *a priori* independent of the other components of θ, with prior specified as uniform over $(0,1)^2$. Then, following (5.3), the limiting posterior distribution on ψ has a stochastic representation as a linear combination of two independent $\operatorname{Unif}(0,1)$ random variables.

Aside: Linear Combinations of Uniforms

A little nuisance arises in calculating the distribution of a linear combination
of uniforms. This is not a sufficiently standard distribution to be listed in most
textbooks, but it is simply characterized. Without loss of generality, say we are
interested in the distribution of $W = U_1 + U_2$, where U_1 and U_2 are independent,
with $U_1 \sim \text{Unif}(0, 1)$ and $U_2 \sim \text{Unif}(0, c)$, with $0 < c < 1$. Appealing to the left
panel of Figure 5.1, we can see geometrically that

$$Pr(W < w) = \begin{cases} c^{-1}(1/2)w^2 & \text{if } w < c; \\ c^{-1}\{(1/2)w^2 - (1/2)(w-c)^2\} & \text{if } c \leq w \leq 1; \\ c^{-1}\{c - (1/2)(1-w+c)^2\} & \text{if } w > c. \end{cases}$$

From here we can differentiate to obtain the density function of W. This results
in a trapezoidal-shaped density function, as depicted in the right panel of Figure 5.1, with base running from 0 to $1 + c$, and top running from c to 1, with
height 1.★

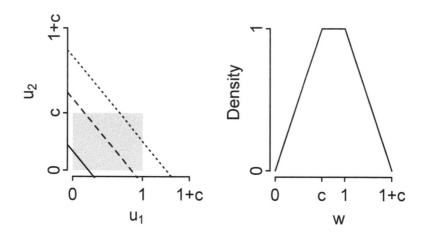

Figure 5.1 *Determining the distribution of a linear combination of two independent
uniform random variables. With reference to the left panel, note that $Pr(W < w)$ is the
portion of the shaded rectangle below the line $u_2 = w - u_1$. This is determined via areas
of triangles for the three cases $0 < w < c$ (i.e., portion below the solid line), $c \leq w \leq 1$
(i.e., portion below the dashed line), and $1 < w < 1 + c$ (i.e., portion below the dotted
line). Differentiating the distribution function then gives the density of W, as depicted
in the right panel.*

Application of the above calculation to our problem is direct, and the properties of the limiting posterior distribution can be summarized as follows.

Following Gustafson (2011), the limiting posterior distribution of the average causal effect ψ has a trapezoidal-shaped density centered at $a(\phi)$. The base of the trapezoid extends over $a(\phi) \pm b(\phi)$, while the top extends over $a(\phi) \pm \tilde{b}(\phi)$, with

$$\tilde{b}(\phi) = \frac{\max\{r_n, r_a\} - \min\{r_n, r_a\}}{2}.$$

Thus the width of the support of the LPD is equal to the proportion of non-compliers in the population, while the peakedness is governed by the mix within the non-compliers. The most peaked situation is the balanced case of $r_n = r_a$, in which case $\tilde{b}(\phi) = 0$, i.e., the LPD has a triangular density. The least peaked situation is the completely imbalanced case of $r_n = 0$ or $r_a = 0$ (but $r_n + r_a > 0$). In this case $\tilde{b}(\phi) = b(\phi)$, i.e., the LPD is a uniform distribution.

Right away we see this is a situation of strong indirect learning where the data "speak loudly." That is, multiple values of ϕ can give rise to the same values of $a(\phi)$ and $b(\phi)$, but different values of $\tilde{b}(\phi)$. So the data have more to say asymptotically than simply telling us the identification region for the target.

Computing the Posterior Distribution

Having characterized the limiting posterior distribution, we turn our attention to finite-sample inference. We start with a uniform prior distribution as $\pi(\theta)$, or more formally a Dirichlet$(1,1,1)$ prior on (r_n, r_a, r_c), and a uniform prior on each p_{ux}, for $u \in \{c,n,a\}$, $x \in \{0,1\}$. To apply importance sampling, we take the marginal convenience prior $\pi^*(\phi)$ as $q_{z\bullet\bullet}^\star \sim$ Dirichlet$(1,1,1,1)$, independently for $z = 0, 1$. This is conjugate, leading to Dirichlet posterior marginal distributions for $q_{z\bullet\bullet}$. We can combine this with taking the conditional convenience prior $\pi^*(p_{n1}, p_{a0}|q)$ to be uniform on $(0,1)^2$. Then it is trivial to sample from the joint convenience posterior, and, in light of (5.2), the importance weights needed to convert from the convenience posterior to the actual posterior simply take the form

$$w \propto \frac{1}{(1 - r_a - r_n)^2 r_a r_n}.$$

Demonstrations

As a first demonstration, we simulate data under the parameter settings $(r_n, r_a) = (0.3, 0.05)$, $p_{c\bullet} = (0.5, 0.7)$, $p_{n\bullet} = (0.3, 0.6)$, $p_{a\bullet} = (0.7, 0.8)$, leading to $\psi = 0.225$. The data are generated via balanced randomization, i.e., $Pr(Z = 1) = 0.5$. This is done for a telescoping data sequence with "stops" at $n = 50$, $n = 200$, and $n = 800$. The resulting posterior distributions on the average causal effect are portrayed in Figure 5.2, along with the prior and limiting posterior distributions for comparison. We see substantial Bayesian updating upon receipt of the first 50 datapoints, and an "identified-like" further concentration upon moving to $n = 200$, i.e., quadrupling the sample size approximately concentrates the posterior by a factor of two. After this, however, it is very much a case of diminishing returns. There is little further updating in going to $n = 800$, and indeed with this much data in hand the posterior marginal distribution is very close to its limit.

We do one further demonstration by keeping all the same parameter settings, except replacing $(r_n, r_a) = (0.3, 0.05)$ with $(r_n, r_a) = (0.19, 0.16)$. This changes the value of the target to $\psi = 0.203$. However, the proportion of noncompliers remains at 0.35, implying that the width of support for the limiting posterior distribution is unchanged. With less imbalance between never-takers and always-takers now, the limiting posterior is more peaked, with its density being almost triangular. Again the posterior distributions arising from a telescoping data sequence are displayed, this time in Figure 5.3. The pattern of concentration with increasing n is much as in Figure 5.2. Further comparing to Figure 5.2, note that the more concentrated shape of the posterior distribution is clear at $n = 200$ and very evident at $n = 800$. Thus the ability of the data to speak to the "shape" of the posterior distribution is manifested in finite samples, not just in the asymptotic limit.■

Aside: Counterfactuals in Causal Inference Models

We mentioned in passing that the Example F model includes parameters that may be scientifically interpretable but cannot be directly linked to empirically manifested quantities. These are p_{n1} and p_{a0}, the chances of a successful outcome respectively for a never-taker who takes treatment and for an always-taker who does not take treatment. In fact, much of the literature on causal inference dwells more upon this point, and models such *counterfactual* situations more explicitly. To say a few words on how this would look in the Example F context, we could explicitly write a *pair* of outcomes for each subject, $(Y^{(0)}, Y^{(1)})$, these being the outcomes that would be seen if the subject does not or does transpire to take treatment. That is, while each subject is thought to have values for $(Z, X, U, Y^{(0)}, Y^{(1)})$, only (Z, X, Y) are observable, where $Y = Y^{(X)} = (1 - X)Y^{(0)} + XY^{(1)}$.

With this formulation, key assumptions about dealing with confounding can then be expressed in terms of conditional independence of the potential outcomes and the treatment indicator. In the present setting, for instance, the assumption that $(Y^{(0)}, Y^{(1)})$ are conditionally independent of X given compli-

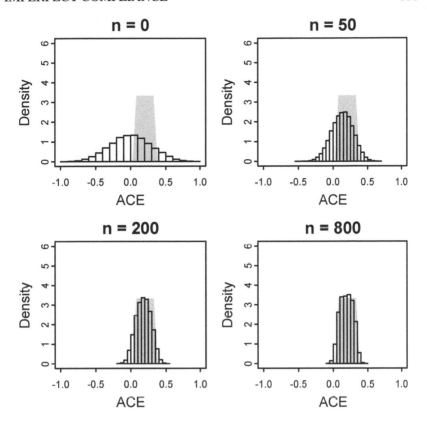

Figure 5.2 *Posterior distribution for the ACE in Example F, as a function of sample size. Synthetic data are generated with "stops" at $n = 50$, $n = 200$, $n = 800$, under parameter values $(r_n, r_a) = (0.3, 0.05)$, $p_{c\bullet} = (0.5, 0.7)$, $p_{n\bullet} = (0.3, 0.6)$, $p_{a\bullet} = (0.7, 0.8)$. The prior (the $n = 0$ panel) and the limiting posterior distribution (shaded density in every panel) are also indicated. The three posterior distributions are determined via importance sampling with 50,000 draws, leading to effective sample sizes ranging from 41,500 ($n = 50$) to 48,600 ($n = 800$).*

ance type U is central, and leads to

$$
\begin{aligned}
E(Y|X = 1, U) &= E\left\{(1 - X)Y^{(0)} + XY^{(1)}|X = 1, U\right\} \\
&= E\left(Y^{(1)}|X = 1, U\right) \\
&= E\left(Y^{(1)}|U\right).
\end{aligned}
$$

Similarly, $E(Y|X = 0, U) = E(Y^{(0)}|U)$. Now recall that the ACE given in (5.1) has the form $E\{E(Y|X = 1, U) - E(Y|X = 0|U)\}$. We now see this as equiv-

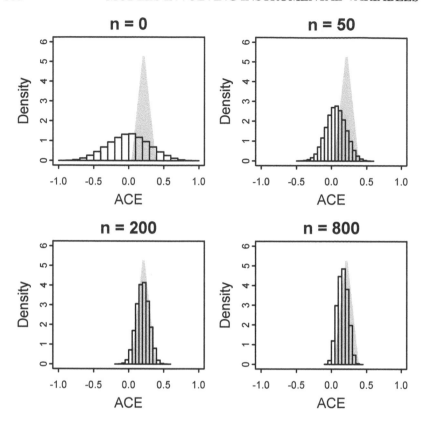

Figure 5.3 *Posterior distribution for the ACE in Example F, as a function of sample size. Synthetic data are generated with "stops" at $n = 50$, $n = 200$, $n = 800$, under parameter values $(r_n, r_a) = (0.19, 0.16)$, $p_{c\bullet} = (0.5, 0.7)$, $p_{n\bullet} = (0.3, 0.6)$, $p_{a\bullet} = (0.7, 0.8)$. The prior ($n = 0$ panel) and the limiting posterior distribution (shaded density in every panel) are also indicated. The three posterior distributions are determined via importance sampling with 50,000 draws, leading to effective sample sizes ranging from 31,800 ($n = 50$) to 49,500 ($n = 800$).*

alent to $E\{E(Y^{(1)}|U) - E(Y^{(0)}|U)\} = E(Y^{(1)} - Y^{(0)})$. The latter form emphasizes that this really is a quantity of causal interest, that can be thought of as contrasting the situation when all population members are treated versus that when none are treated. ★

5.3 Modeling an Approximate Instrumental Variable

Generally IV assumptions (ii) and (iii) cannot be verified or falsified empirically, since they pertain to an unobservable variable U. In applications then, particularly in the biostatistical sphere, whether or not a putative instrumental variable really satisfies the assumptions can be an article of faith. For this reason, it is worth considering what happens if we replace one of the conditional independence assumptions with a weaker assumption, namely that any conditional dependence is likely to be mild. This harkens back to Chapter 3, and the tradeoff between invoking a sharp assumption to gain identification at the cost of possible model misspecification, versus invoking a fuzzier assumption that does not induce identification. Indeed, there was mention in Section 3.5 of Gustafson (2007) which involves an instrumental variable, but in the context of dealing with a mismeasured variable rather than an unobserved variable. The essence of that work is to weaken an assumption analogous to the present assumption (iii). We now adapt this approach to the present context of dealing with confounding arising from an unobserved variable.

Example G: Weakening an Instrumental Variable Assumption

Now we turn our attention to a normal linear model structure for a response variable of interest Y, an exposure of interest X, a possible instrumental variable Z, and an unobservable confounding variable U. The model is

$$
\begin{aligned}
Y|X,U,Z &\sim N(\beta_0 + \beta_x X + \beta_u U + \beta_z Z, \sigma^2), \\
X|U,Z &\sim N(\alpha_0 + \alpha_u U + \alpha_z Z, \tau^2), \\
U|Z &\sim N(0,1).
\end{aligned}
$$

This nine parameter model, with

$$
\theta = (\beta_0, \beta_x, \beta_z, \beta_u, \alpha_0, \alpha_z, \alpha_u, \sigma^2, \tau^2), \tag{5.4}
$$

completely specifies the distribution of $(Y, X, U|Z)$, and hence the distribution of $(Y, X|Z)$, with the latter being learnable from the data. Note also that one of the IV assumptions, that U and Z are independent of one another, is already "hard-wired" into the above model specification. The other two assumptions can be expressed as suppositions about parameter values within the model. First, the assumption that exposure is associated with the IV given confounders corresponds to $\alpha_z \neq 0$. Second, the assumption that outcome and IV are conditionally independent given confounders corresponds to $\beta_z = 0$. Finally, note that since U is not observed, it can be scaled arbitrarily. So, the assumption that U has mean zero and variance one is without loss of generality. By the same token, the sign of U is arbitrary. So we also assume, without loss of generality, that $\alpha_u \geq 0$.

A standard instrumental variable analysis would assume $\beta_z = 0$, i.e., the instrument has no direct influence on the outcome. We consider situations where this assumption might be debatable, and a more defensible assumption would be that β_z is unlikely to be large in magnitude. Or, more to the point, the user would willingly commit to a prior distribution quantifying a threshold beyond which $|\beta_z|$ is unlikely to fall.

Transparent Parameterization

Toward a transparent parameterization for this problem, let γ be a 2×2 matrix of parameters, let κ be a 2×1 vector of parameters, and let Ω be a 2×2 covariance matrix, such that

$$\begin{pmatrix} Y \\ X \end{pmatrix} Z,U \Bigg) \sim N_2 \left\{ (\gamma \; \kappa) \begin{pmatrix} 1 \\ Z \\ U \end{pmatrix}, \Omega \right\}.$$

Standard bivariate normal distribution theory applied to the initial model structure gives us

$$(\gamma \; \kappa) = \left[\begin{array}{c} (\beta_0 \; \beta_z \; \beta_u) + \beta_x(\alpha_0 \; \alpha_z \; \alpha_u) \\ (\alpha_0 \; \alpha_z \; \alpha_u) \end{array} \right],$$

and

$$\Omega = \begin{pmatrix} \sigma^2 + \beta_x^2 \tau^2 & \beta_x \tau^2 \\ & \tau^2 \end{pmatrix}.$$

As a next step, we then have

$$\begin{pmatrix} Y \\ X \end{pmatrix} Z \Bigg) \sim N_2 \left\{ \gamma \begin{pmatrix} 1 \\ Z \end{pmatrix}, \Sigma \right\}, \tag{5.5}$$

where

$$\Sigma = \Omega + \kappa \kappa^T.$$

Now, (5.5) suggests that $\phi = (\gamma, \Sigma)$ and $\lambda = \kappa$ could serve as a transparent parameterization, with $\dim(\phi) = 7$ and $\dim(\lambda) = 2$. To verify that the map from θ to (γ, Σ, κ) is invertible, note that we can apply the following, in turn:

$$\begin{aligned}
\tau^2 &= (\Sigma - \kappa \kappa^T)_{22} \\
\beta_x &= (\Sigma - \kappa \kappa^T)_{12} / \tau^2 \\
\sigma^2 &= \Sigma - \kappa \kappa^T)_{11} - \beta_x \tau^2 \\
(\alpha_0, \alpha_z, \alpha_u) &= (\gamma \; \kappa)_{2\bullet} \\
(\beta_0, \beta_z, \beta_u) &= (\gamma \; \kappa)_{1\bullet} - \beta_x(\alpha_0, \alpha_z, \alpha_u).
\end{aligned}$$

Determining the Identification Region

To express the identification region in this framework, note that for given $\phi = (\gamma, \Sigma)$, the inverse mapping will bring us back to the original parameter space so long as (i) $\kappa_2 \geq 0$, and (ii) $\Sigma - \kappa \kappa^T$ is positive definite. The second requirement is equivalent to

$$\kappa^T \Sigma^{-1} \kappa \leq 1, \tag{5.6}$$

allowing us to visualize the identification region as the interior of a half-ellipse in the (κ_1, κ_2) plane.

To give an example, consider the values of γ and Σ which arise when the underlying true parameter values are $(\alpha_0, \alpha_z, \alpha_u) = (0, 0.5, 0.25)$, $(\beta_0, \beta_x, \beta_z, \beta_u) = (0, 0.75, 0, -0.25)$, $\sigma = 1$, $\tau = 1$. The resulting identification region for κ is depicted in the left panel of Figure 5.4. Superimposed on the identification region are contours corresponding to fixed values of β_z, obtained upon noting that the inverse mapping gives

$$\beta_z = \gamma_{21} - \gamma_{22} \left(\frac{\Sigma_{12} - \kappa_1 \kappa_2}{\Sigma_{22} - \kappa_2^2} \right).$$

From here we immediately see that the data themselves do not rule out any values of β_z, i.e., for all b the curve corresponding to $\beta_z = b$ intersects the identification region. This confirms the futility of attempting the problem unless an *a priori* assumption about the magnitude of β_z is justified.

It should also be pointed out that *a posteriori* uncertainty about β_z transmutes directly to uncertainty about the parameter of interest, β_x. Again with $\phi = (\gamma, \Sigma)$ fixed, β_x is determined from β_z as

$$\beta_x = \frac{\gamma_{12} - \beta_z}{\gamma_{22}}.$$

Hence the limiting posterior variance of β_x will be $\gamma_{22}^{-2} = \alpha_z^{-2}$ times the limiting posterior variance of β_z. This is a version of the "instrument strength" argument seen in the identified case, whereby a stronger association between exposure X and instrument Z, as reflected by a larger value of $|\alpha_z|$, leads to sharper inference on the conditional (X, Y) association.

Now we turn our attention to situations where an assumption that β_z is small can be imposed. As a reminder, this corresponds to the supposition that Z is *nearly* an instrumental variable. Consider the situation of imposing the prior distribution $\beta_z \sim \text{Unif}(-\varepsilon, \varepsilon)$. From the geometry of Figure 5.4, it is clear that such hard *a priori* bounds on β_z will reduce the identification region for κ, i.e., we end up with only the portion of the half-ellipse that falls between the $\beta_z = -\varepsilon$ contour and the $\beta_z = \varepsilon$ contour.

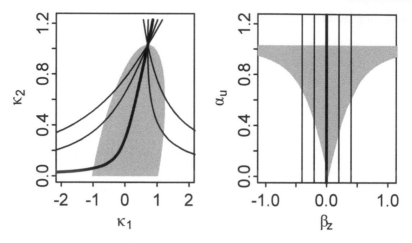

Figure 5.4 *The identification region in Example G, for the values of (γ, Σ) given in the text. The shaded half-ellipse in the left panel gives the region in terms of κ, with the superimposed curves being contours for $\beta_z = 0$ (thicker curve), $\beta_z = \pm 0.2$ and $\beta_z = \pm 0.4$. The right panel gives the identification region and these contours transformed into the (β_z, α_u) plane.*

Determining the Limiting Posterior Distribution

While the geometric interpretation above is helpful for visualization purposes, it is less helpful for computing the limiting posterior distribution. In applying the importance sampling strategy for LPDs outlined in Chapter 2, we need to draw samples from a proposal distribution for $(\kappa|\gamma, \Sigma)$, with the support of this distribution containing the identification region. The scheme is only efficient, however, if the support of the proposal distribution is not too much bigger than the identification region. And the geometrical picture in the left panel of Figure 5.4 does not inspire an obvious choice of proposal distribution.

We instead proceed by further reparameterizing the problem. For fixed $\phi = (\gamma, \Sigma)$ it is clear that the map from κ to

$$
\begin{pmatrix} \beta_z \\ \alpha_u \end{pmatrix} = \begin{pmatrix} \gamma_{12} - \gamma_{22}(\Sigma_{12} - \kappa_1 \kappa_2)/(\Sigma_{22} - \kappa_2^2) \\ \kappa_2 \end{pmatrix}
$$

is invertible. Hence, the map from θ to $(\gamma, \Sigma, \beta_z, \alpha_u)$ must also constitute a transparent parameterization for this problem. In our running example, the right panel of Figure 5.4 shows the identification region in the (β_z, α_u) plane, i.e., the right panel depicts the transform of the region in the left panel.

So we now pursue the transparent parameterization $\phi = (\gamma, \Sigma)$, $\lambda = (\beta_z, \alpha_u)$. While the boundary of the identification region in this parameterization is somewhat messy to characterize, from (5.6) we do inherit marginally the constraint $0 < \alpha_u < \Sigma_{22}^{1/2}$. It is also possible to directly calculate the Jacobian term for this map, obtaining

$$\left| \frac{\partial(\phi \; \lambda)}{\partial \theta} \right| \;\; = \;\; |\alpha_z \alpha_u|.$$

So we proceed with the importance sampling approach to computing the LPD, taking the proposal distribution to be a uniform distribution on the rectangle of the form $(\beta_z, \alpha_u) \in (-\varepsilon, \varepsilon) \times \left(0, \Sigma_{22}^{1/2} \right)$. From the geometric considerations in the right panel of Figure 5.4, we see that the support of this proposal distribution strictly contains the identification region. Hence some sampled points will receive zero weight. Specifically, we can express the importance weights as

$$w(\beta_z, \alpha_u) \;\; = \;\; \pi(\theta(\gamma^\dagger, \Sigma^\dagger, \beta_z, \alpha_u)) |\alpha_u|^{-1} I_{R(\gamma^\dagger, \Sigma^\dagger)}(\beta_z, \alpha_u),$$

regarding $\phi = \phi^\dagger$ as true values, and using $R(\gamma, \Sigma)$ to indicate the identification region for (β_z, α_u).

Continuing our example, say that the prior distribution $\pi(\theta)$ is comprised of independent components, with the $N(0, 10^2)$ distribution assigned to each of the six regression coefficients other than β_z, and the $IG(0.1, 0.1)$ distribution assigned to both of the variance components. This constitutes a very weakly informative prior. Figure 5.5 gives results of the importance sampling algorithm applied to the $(\gamma^\dagger, \Sigma^\dagger)$ values used for Figure 5.4 in tandem with the *a priori* bound based on $\varepsilon = 0.25$. The bivariate posterior distributions of (κ_1, κ_2) (upper-left panel) and (β_z, α_u) (upper-right panel) can be compared to Figure 5.4, to assess the impact of the *a priori* bound on β_z. Unsurprisingly, the limiting posterior support of β_z is seen to be the same as the prior support, speaking to the role of ε as a sensitivity parameter. However, the limiting posterior distribution on β_z is somewhat more peaked than the uniform prior, reflecting some limited Bayesian updating. As already described, the limiting posterior on the target of inference β_x is a linear transformation of the limiting posterior on β_z. Note that in this particular example the true value of the target, $\beta_x^\dagger = 0.75$, lies at the center of the limiting posterior distribution. This arises since $\beta_z^\dagger = 0$ happens to lie at the center of the corresponding prior distribution.

To further consider the LPD in this problem, we fix $(\beta_0, \beta_x, \beta_u)^\dagger = (0, 0.75, -0.25)$, $(\alpha_0, \alpha_u)^\dagger = (0, 0.25)$, $\sigma^\dagger = 1$, and $\tau^\dagger = 1$. Then we consider all values of $\phi^\dagger$ arising from combinations of (i) $\alpha_z^\dagger \in \{0.4, 0.8\}$, and (ii) $\beta_z^\dagger \in \{-0.2, -0.1, 0, 0.1, 0.2\}$. Again the prior specification is based on the $N(0, 10^2)$ distribution for each regression coefficient other than β_z and the $IG(0.1, 0.1)$ for both variance components. Now, however, the bounding value for β_z a priori is $\varepsilon = 0.15$. Note that in considering these two different values of $\alpha_z^\dagger$, we are studying the impact of having a weaker or stronger instrument. And the five values of $\beta_z^\dagger$ range from outside to inside the $\pm \varepsilon$ *a priori* bound.

The LPDs for β_x, as determined by importance sampling, are depicted in

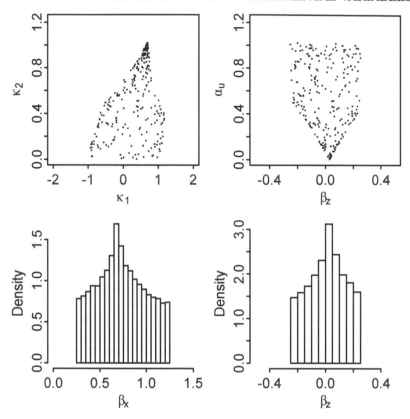

Figure 5.5 *The limiting posterior distribution in Example G, for the values of* (γ, Σ) *given in the text. This was computed from a Monte Carlo sample size of* 10^5, *resulting in 76,300 points with positive weight and an effective sample size of 29,700. The bivariate scatterplots arise from sampling 250 points according to the importance weights.*

Figure 5.6, via tri-interval plots. Note first that we see the sort of calibration we might expect: the 95% HPD interval for β_x contains the true value for precisely those settings where the true value $\beta_z^\dagger$ lies inside the prior interval. Second, note that the LPDs are extremely skewed in some cases, particularly when the true value $\beta_z^\dagger$ falls outside the prior interval. Third, note that the impact of instrument strength is very evident. As per our earlier mathematical argument, we do indeed see that a doubling of $|\alpha_z|$ induces a halving of the width of the LPD.

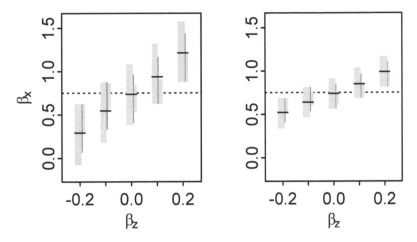

Figure 5.6 *The limiting posterior distribution of β_x in Example G, when $\alpha_z = 0.4$ (left panel) and $\alpha_z = 0.8$ (right panel), under various values of β_z. The a priori bound is $|\beta_z| < 0.15$. Other parameter values and hyperparameter settings are described in the text. Each LPD is determined using importance sampling with 100,000 draws. In all ten settings, the number of draws receiving positive weight exceeds 53,000. The lowest of the effective sample sizes is 3,000 (for $\alpha_z = 0.8, \beta_z = 0.1$), and the second lowest is 14,000 (for $\alpha_z = 0.4, \beta_z = -0.1$).*

Determining the Posterior Distribution

As with other examples we have seen, we wish to leverage our algorithm for computing the LPD into an algorithm for computing the finite-sample posterior distribution. Doing so necessitates choosing a convenience prior marginal $\pi^*(\gamma, \Sigma)$ and conditional $\pi^*(\beta_z, \alpha_s | \gamma, \Sigma)$. The latter specification can be the same uniform distribution used in the LPD computation. The former can be chosen to facilitate Monte Carlo sampling of $\pi^*(\gamma, \Sigma | d_n)$. Taking γ and Σ to be *a priori* independently distributed according to a normal distribution and inverse Wishart distribution fits this bill. This leads to an easy Gibbs sampling algorithm for MCMC sampling of $\pi^*(\gamma, \Sigma | d_n)$.

Aside: Markov Chain Monte Carlo Details

The bivariate structure of (5.5) leads to somewhat more messy posterior structure than is seen with normal linear regression models for a univariate response. Nonetheless, the same ideas apply. For instance, if we consider stacking the two rows of γ as a vector, then, as a function of γ with d_n and Σ fixed,

$$\pi(d_n | \gamma, \Sigma) \quad \propto \quad \exp\{(-1/2)(\gamma^T A \gamma - 2B^T \gamma)\},$$

where

$$A = \sum_{i=1}^{n} \Sigma^{-1} \otimes \begin{pmatrix} 1 & z_i \\ z_i & z_i^2 \end{pmatrix},$$

and

$$B = \sum_{i=1}^{n} \text{vec} \left[\Sigma^{-1} \begin{pmatrix} y_i & y_i z_i \\ x_i & x_i z_i \end{pmatrix} \right]^T.$$

From here, it is straightforward but tedious "bookkeeping" for normal linear forms to deduce the multivariate normal distribution of $\pi(\gamma | \Sigma, d_n)$. Similarly, for fixed γ and d_n we have

$$\pi(d_n | \gamma, \Sigma) \propto |\Sigma^{-1}|^{n/2} \exp\left(-(1/2) \sum_{i=1}^{n} w_i^T \Sigma^{-1} w_i \right),$$

where

$$w_i = \begin{pmatrix} y_i \\ x_i \end{pmatrix} - \gamma \begin{pmatrix} 1 \\ z_i \end{pmatrix}.$$

From this point it is straightforward, but again tedious, to determine the inverse Wishart distribution of $\pi(\Sigma | \gamma, d_n)$. ★

Armed with our MCMC-based sample from the convenience posterior distribution, importance reweighting to achieve the actual posterior is based on the weighting scheme

$$w(\gamma, \Sigma, \beta_z, \alpha_u) = \frac{\pi(\theta(\gamma, \Sigma, \beta_z, \alpha_u)) |\gamma_{22} \alpha_u|^{-1}}{\pi^*(\gamma) \pi^*(\Sigma) \pi^*(\beta_z, \alpha_u | \Sigma)}.$$

Here, since the support of the proposal distribution is larger than that of the target, it is understood that points not in the image of the reparameterization to $(\gamma, \Sigma, \beta_z, \alpha_u)$ get zero weight.

Demonstration

We generate three synthetic (Y, X, Z) datasets of size $n = 400$ under one of the settings used above in Figure 5.6, namely $(\beta_0, \beta_x, \beta_z, \beta_u)^\dagger = (0, 0.75, 0.1, -0.25)$, $(\alpha_0, \alpha_x, \alpha_u)^\dagger = (0, 0.8, 0.25)$, $\sigma^\dagger = 1$, and $\tau^\dagger = 1$. Because the computation is slower and more intricate than in other examples (using MCMC *and* importance sampling rather than just importance sampling), we use the naïve strategy of computing each posterior distribution twice using independent MCMC runs. This is just a simple-minded check on whether

Monte Carlo error is controlled. We do this particularly as the effective sample size obtained from the importance weights is a less useful gauge when the original sample is not independent and identically distributed.

Results, in the form of tri-interval plots for β_x, appear in Figure 5.7. The LPD, exactly as per Figure 5.6, is also portrayed for comparison. We do see (i) stability across the two MCMC runs, (ii) modest sampling variability in the posterior distributions, and (iii) posterior distributions which are only slightly wider than the LPD. This is very much in keeping with the behavior we have seen in other examples throughout this book.■

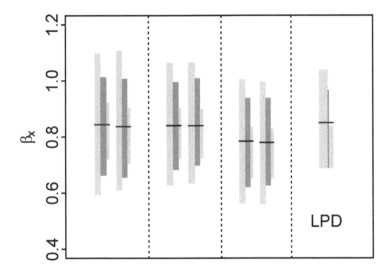

Figure 5.7 *The posterior distribution of β_x in Example G, arising from three synthetic datasets of size n = 400. The parameter settings underlying the data generation are given in full in the text, and correspond to the case of $\alpha_z = 0.8$, $\beta_z - 0.1$ in Figure 5.6. For each dataset, the posterior is computed twice via the combination of MCMC and importance sampling described in the text, using 20,000 MCMC iterations following 1,000 burn-in iterations. The number of points attracting non-zero weight ranges from 2,900 to 3,700 across the six posterior computations. For comparison, the LPD as given in Figure 5.6 is also depicted.*

Chapter 6

Further Examples

6.1 Inference in the Face of a Hidden Subpopulation

A fairly common challenge in using samples to infer properties of populations is that some of the population may be inaccessible or "closed-off" to sampling. For instance, say the population of interest is all adults in a geographic jurisdiction, but the sampling proceeds via telephone calls to "landline" phone numbers. Then the portion of the population not having landlines will be inaccessible. The challenge can become particularly acute when dealing with so-called "hard-to-reach" populations, for which most forms of probability-based sampling are difficult, if not impossible, to implement. Examples of hard-to-reach populations include populations defined by illicit drug use, and populations defined by sexual behaviors. There is considerable recent literature on both sampling hard-to-reach populations and appropriately analyzing the resulting data. Some prominent sampling schemes include "respondent-driven sampling," "snowball sampling," and "venue sampling." As a few recent entry points into this literature, see Gile and Handcock (2010), Johnston and Sabin (2010), Semaan (2010), Karon and Wejnert (2012), and Gustafson et al. (2013).

Typical schemes to sample from hard-to-reach populations tend to involve some population members having a higher chance than others of being recruited into the sample. If the investigator has information on these selection probabilities, for those who happen to be recruited into the sample, then there is hope of valid statistical adjustment. Technically, this is achieved via the use of *sampling weights*, whereby data from sample members who actually had *less* chance of being sampled carry *more* weight in the analysis. Very often, however, the sampling scheme will have a further deficiency: some population members have zero chance of being recruited into the sample. These population members constitute the inaccessible subpopulation. And, as we shall see, the presence of an inaccessible subpopulation can push us from the identified model context to the partially identified context.

Example H: Prevalence Estimation with a Hidden Subpopulation

Let the observable Y be a unit's binary trait of interest, while the observable $Q \geq 0$ is proportional to a unit's selection probability. That is, a population member with $Q = a$ is a/b times more likely to be recruited into the sample than a population member with $Q = b$. And we explicitly acknowledge that the population of interest may have an inaccessible component, in the form of population members with $Q = 0$.

Following Xia and Gustafson (2012), we model the *observed* realizations of (Y, Q) as *iid* realizations of (Y, Q) from the bivariate density $f(y, q)$. But we must then be careful to distinguish this density from the bivariate density that describes the distribution of (Y, Q) across the target population. Since part of the population is inaccessible, and since the observed data arise from a weighted sampling scheme, the density *actually describing* the target population is

$$f^*(y,q) \quad = \quad (1-p)\frac{q^{-1}f(y,q)}{\int_0^\infty \tilde{q}^{-1}\{f(0,\tilde{q}) + f(1,\tilde{q})\}\,d\tilde{q}} + p\delta_0(q)f(y|0), (6.1)$$

where p is the proportion of the target population that is inaccessible, while $\delta_0()$ denotes a point-mass distribution at zero.

We parameterize $f(y, q)$ by (α, β), such that

$$f(y|q) \quad = \quad \{\mu(q;\beta)\}^y \{1 - \mu(q;\beta)\}^{1-y}, \tag{6.2}$$

i.e., $E_f(Y|Q) = Pr_f(Y = 1|Q) = \mu(Q;\beta)$. And the marginal distribution of Q is expressed as $f(q; \alpha)$. So the initial parameterization of our problem can be taken as $\theta = (\alpha, \beta, p)$. Moreover, this trivially cleaves into a transparent parameterization, with $\phi = (\alpha, \beta)$ describing the joint distribution of the observables, while $\lambda = p$ does not appear in the likelihood function.

While the transparent parameterization is very simple in this problem, the target of inference depends on the parameters in quite a complicated manner. To wit, the prevalence of Y in the target population is the mean of Y according to (6.1), expressed as

$$\psi \quad = \quad (1-p)\frac{\int q^{-1}\mu(q;\beta)f(q;\alpha)\,dq}{\int q^{-1}f(q;\alpha)\,dq} + p\mu(0;\beta). \tag{6.3}$$

In particular, we already sense that at best we can hope for partial information about this target, since it depends non-trivially on both $\phi = (\alpha, \beta)$ and $\lambda = p$.

Before proceeding, we pause to comment on a rather strong assumption embedded in (6.2) and (6.3). The prevalence of Y in the inaccessible subpopulation is presumed to be $\mu(0;\beta) = \lim_{q\downarrow 0}\mu(q;\beta)$, This is a key assumption, which views the inaccessible subpopulation (defined by $Q = 0$) as the limit of ever harder-to-reach subpopulations (defined by Q decreasing to zero). The appropriateness of this continuity assumption will be context-specific. For instance, say the weighted scheme results from venue sampling, whereby population members are sampled at venues where they tend to congregate, so that larger values of Q correspond to more frequent attendance at these venues.

Then the continuity assumption devolves to an assumption that never-attenders are the limiting case of seldom-attenders, which may be quite reasonable.

Determining the Limited Posterior Distribution

To deconstruct inference in this setting, we denote the trait prevalances amongst the accessible and inaccessible (or "hidden") subpopulations as

$$\psi_{acc}(\alpha,\beta) = \frac{\int q^{-1}\mu(q;\beta)f(q;\alpha)\,dq}{\int q^{-1}f(q;\alpha)\,dq}$$

and

$$\psi_{hid}(\beta) = \mu(0;\beta)$$

respectively. Clearly these are identified quantities. Moreover, they lead us to a simple characterization of the limiting posterior distribution of the target parameter (6.3).

The limiting posterior distribution of ψ has a stochastic representation as

$$\psi^\star = \psi_{acc}\left(\alpha^\dagger,\beta^\dagger\right) + \left\{\psi_{hid}\left(\beta^\dagger\right) - \psi_{acc}\left(\alpha^\dagger,\beta^\dagger\right)\right\}p^\star, \qquad (6.4)$$

where $p^\star$ is distributed according to the conditional prior density $\pi(p|\alpha^\dagger,\beta^\dagger)$. Consequently, the uncertainty that remains about the target as the data accumulate is readily characterized by

$$\mathrm{Var}(\psi^\star|d_n) \rightarrow \left\{\psi_{hid}\left(\beta^\dagger\right) - \psi_{acc}\left(\alpha^\dagger,\beta^\dagger\right)\right\}^2 \times$$
$$\mathrm{Var}\{p^\star|(\alpha^\star,\beta^\star) = (\alpha^\dagger,\beta^\dagger)\},$$

as n goes to infinity.

   In fact, the situation will typically be even simpler than described above. There is no compelling link between prior information about the proportion of the population that is inaccessible and the prior information about the distribution of (Y,Q) in the accessible subpopulation. Therefore, a priori independence of the form $\pi(p,\alpha,\beta) = \pi(p)\pi(\alpha,\beta)$ would typically be assumed. In this case, the characterization shows directly how the specified prior information for p propagates through to inference about the target parameter.

Demonstration

To demonstrate inference in this model, we simulate data under the following conditions. For simplicity we take Q to be discrete, with "observable" support

$Q \in \{1, \ldots, 10\}$ (but of course $Q = 0$ for units in the inaccessible subpopulation). Then we can simply define $\alpha_i = Pr(Q = i)$, for $i = 1, \ldots, 10$, with $\sum_{i=1}^{10} \alpha_i = 1$ necessarily. We take the $(Y|Q)$ relationship to be governed by

$$\text{logit } \mu(q; \beta) \quad = \quad \beta_0 + \beta_1 q + \beta_1 q^2.$$

This simple quadratic relationship is assumed just for the sake of illustration. For real applications there would be more advisable choices for modeling a smooth dependence of Y on Q. Particularly, Xia and Gustafson (2012) consider using splines for this purpose.

The prior assigned to p is the Beta$(6, 24)$ distribution, which has mean 0.2, and places 97% of its mass between 0.05 and 0.35. A diffuse trivariate normal prior distribution is assigned to $\beta = (\beta_0, \beta_1, \beta_2)$, with mean vector $(0, 0, 0)$ and covariance matrix $25I_3$. And a Dirichlet$(1, 1, \ldots, 1)$ prior is assigned to $\alpha = (\alpha_1, \ldots, \alpha_{10})$. Inference is very easily implemented via importance sampling with a proposal density of the form $\pi^*(\alpha, \beta, p|d_n) = \pi^*(\alpha|d_n)\pi^*(\beta|d_n)\pi^*(p)$. Here we take $\pi^*(\alpha|d_n)$ to be the conjugate Dirichlet posterior distribution based on the observed Q frequencies, we take $\pi^*(\beta|d_n)$ to be the normal distribution with mean and covariance matrix taken as the mode and inverse Hessian of the log-likelihood function from the logistic regression of Y on $(1, Q, Q^2)$, and finally we take $\pi^*(p)$ to be the prior density. Since the contributions of the data to the posterior density and the importance sampling proposal cancel either exactly (in the case of the α term), or approximately (in the case of the β term), this is an efficient algorithm that typically exhibits only very modest variation in the importance weights.

A first set of results arises from data simulated under $\alpha_i^\dagger = i/55$, for $i = 1, \ldots, 10$, and $\beta^\dagger = [\text{logit}(0.2), \{\text{logit}(0.3) - \text{logit}(0.2)\}/10, 0]$. Note that this $\alpha^\dagger$ actually arises from a uniform distribution of Q across the accessible population. As well, this $\beta^\dagger$ corresponds to quite modest association between Y and Q, with the prevalence of Y ranging from 0.2 in the hidden subpopulation to 0.3 in the very likeliest to participate ($Q = 10$) subpopulation.

Posterior inferences for ψ from three independent, "telescoping" data sequences are displayed in Figure 6.1, with the LPD also depicted. A consequence of the modest dependence between Y and Q is that ψ_{acc} and ψ_{hid} are close together, implying a very narrow LPD. Even at quite large sample sizes then, there is further posterior concentration upon further data acquisition. Indeed, the pattern in Figure 6.1 could be mistaken for one involving identified inference, with quadrupling the sample size approximately halving the width of the posterior.

The next set of results, appearing in Figure 6.2, are based on the same settings as above, except with $\alpha^\dagger$ modified. In particular, we take

$$\alpha_i^\dagger \quad = \quad \frac{i \min\{i, 11 - i\}^3}{c},$$

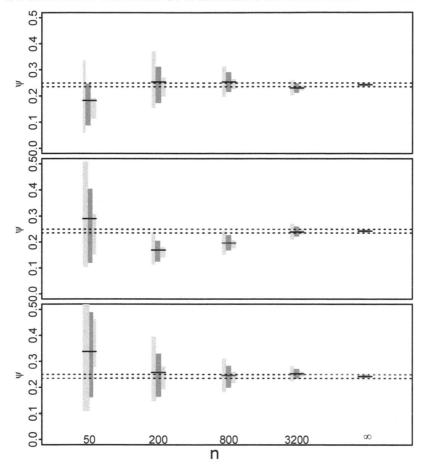

Figure 6.1 *Finite-sample evolution of the posterior marginal distribution of trait preva-*
lence in Example H, for three independent telescoping data sequences. As described in
the text, the underlying value of $\alpha^\dagger$ corresponds to a more variable distribution of Q,
and the underlying value of $\beta^\dagger$ corresponds to weaker association between Q and Y.
For reference, the dashed horizontal lines mark the 95% HPD interval for the limiting
posterior distribution.

with c chosen to ensure that the components of $\alpha^\dagger$ sum to one. This corresponds to the actual distribution of Q in the accessible population being sym-
metrically distributed over $\{1, \ldots, 10\}$, with a very peaked probability mass
function proportional to $\min\{i, 11 - i\}^3$. With less variability in Q than before,
we conjecture that it would be harder to estimate $\psi_{hid} = \mu(0; \beta)$ well. That
is, this estimation now requires more extrapolation from where the bulk of the

Q data reside. However, in comparing Figure 6.2 to Figure 6.1, we are hard-pressed to see a resulting impact in terms of wider posterior distributions.

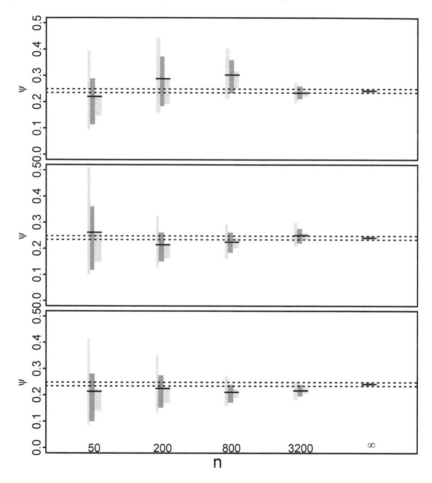

Figure 6.2 *Finite-sample evolution of the posterior marginal distribution of trait preva-lence in Example H, for three independent telescoping data sequences. As described in the text, the underlying value of $\alpha^\dagger$ corresponds to a less variable distribution of Q, and the underlying value of $\beta^\dagger$ corresponds to weaker association between Q and Y. For reference, the dashed horizontal lines mark the 95% HPD interval for the limiting posterior distribution.*

The third and fourth sets of results, in Figures 6.3 and 6.4, use the same values of $\alpha^\dagger$ as in Figures 6.1 and 6.2, respectively. So again they correspond to situations where the actual distribution of Q in the target population is more or less variable. However, the association between Q and Y is now considerably stronger, with

$$\beta^\dagger \;\; = \;\; [\mathrm{logit}(0.05), \{logit(0.45) - logit(0.05)\}/10, 0].$$

Thus there is a ninefold increase in trait prevalence between the most-likely-to-be-sampled subpopulation and the inaccessible subpopulation. This induces a much wider LPD than previously, and consequently we see behavior that is more typical of partial identification. As the sample size grows, we rather quickly see diminishing returns in terms of further reduction in posterior width. Also, note that again we are hard-pressed to see a distinct change in behavior between Figures 6.3 and 6.4. Any increased uncertainty that results from the need to further extrapolate more when the distribution of Q is more concentrated seems to be dwarfed by the other uncertainties at hand.∎

Pure Bias Parameters

Reflecting upon (6.4), we see a somewhat simpler structure than in other partially identified models we have encountered. The parameter p is central, in that its prior distribution drives the posterior distribution of the target parameter. This prompts a definition.

Say (ϕ, λ) is a transparent parameterization with $\dim(\lambda) = 1$, and, in the language of Section 2.2, for the chosen prior π the parameterization is factorable. Or, put more simply, ϕ and λ are *a priori* independent. And say that the inferential focus is on the target parameter $\psi = g(\phi, \lambda)$. If, for every ϕ, $g(\phi, \cdot)$ is a monotone function, then we say λ is a *pure bias parameter*.

An immediate consequence of the definition is as follows. If the true value of a pure bias parameter happens to lie at the a-th quantile of its marginal prior distribution $\pi(\lambda | \phi^\dagger)$, then the true value of the target parameter must lie at either the a-th or $(1 - a)$-th quantile of its limiting posterior distribution. Or, put more colloquially, the "appropriateness" of the limiting posterior distribution of the target as a summary of the truth will exactly equal the appropriateness of the prior distribution of the pure bias parameter as a summary of the truth.

Now Example H is indeed a problem for which *a priori* independence of $\phi = (\alpha, \beta)$ and $\lambda = p$ makes sense. There is no reason to think an expert's *a priori* judgment about the extent to which the population is inaccessible would be linked to judgments about the distribution of (Y, Q) in the accessible subpopulation. So, the marginal prior distribution of the pure bias parameter p will be critical. The narrowness of the posterior distribution on the target will largely be driven by the narrowness of this prior, and the "correctness" of the

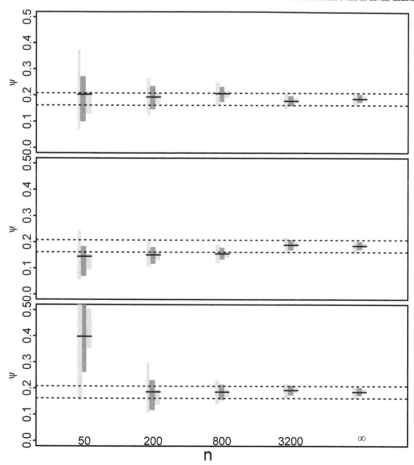

Figure 6.3 *Finite-sample evolution of the posterior marginal distribution of trait preva-*
lence in Example H, for three independent telescoping data sequences. As described in
the text, the underlying value of $\alpha^{\dagger}$ *corresponds to a less variable distribution of Q,*
and the underlying value of $\beta^{\dagger}$ *corresponds to stronger association between Q and Y.*
For reference, the dashed horizontal lines mark the 95% HPD interval for the limiting
posterior distribution.

posterior distribution on the target will largely be driven by the correctness of
this prior distribution. For instance, extending the implications of the pure bias
definition somewhat further, as the sample size goes to infinity, an equal-tailed
95% posterior credible interval for ψ will cover the truth if and only if the
equal-tailed 95% prior credible interval for p covers the truth.

In fact, in this book we have seen other examples that at least *could* in-

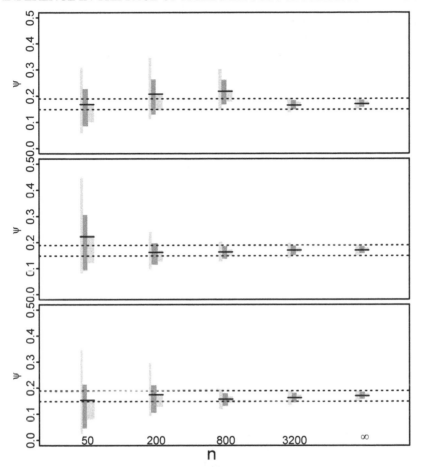

Figure 6.4 *Finite-sample evolution of the posterior marginal distribution of trait prevalence in Example H, for three independent telescoping data sequences. As described in the text, the underlying value of $\alpha^\dagger$ corresponds to a more variable distribution of Q, and the underlying value of $\beta^\dagger$ corresponds to stronger association between Q and Y. For reference, the dashed horizontal lines mark the 95% HPD interval for the limiting posterior distribution.*

volve a pure bias parameter. For instance, consider Example B from Chapter 3. For given ϕ, the target $\psi = Pr(Y = 1)$ as given in (3.4) is monotone in $\lambda = \gamma_{10} = Pr(Y = 1 | X = 1, R = 0)$. (Recall that $R = 0$ indicates missingness, which suggests that indeed γ_{10} is not informed by data.) Moreover, ϕ and λ are variation independent in this problem, meaning at least it would be possible to assign a prior distribution under which ϕ and λ are independent, forcing

λ to be a pure bias parameter. However, the prior actually used in the Example B demonstrations involved independence assumptions that are natural in the original parameterization but induce dependence between ϕ and λ. Hence under this prior λ is not a pure bias parameter.

In another direction, sometimes quantities we might intuit to be pure bias parameters, are, in fact, not. For instance, some elaborations on Example H are given in Xia and Gustafson (2014). One of these involves inferring a relative risk rather than a prevalence, i.e., the interest parameter is $Pr(Y = 1|X = 1)/Pr(Y = 1|X = 0)$, when X and Y are both binary. And now smooth relationships are assumed in q for both $(X|Q = q)$ and $(Y|X, Q = q)$. As before, it is very easy to split the parameters in a transparent fashion. We just take $\lambda = p = Pr(Q = 0)$ and ϕ to be all the other parameters, i.e., all the parameters governing $(X|Q)$ and $(Y|X, Q)$. Again a prior which specifies independence between ϕ and λ would be quite natural, and again the limiting posterior distribution of the target parameter can be represented as a transformation of the prior distribution of p. What Xia and Gustafson (2014) find, however, is that for *some* values of ϕ this transformation is not monotone. So it is no longer guaranteed that the extent to which p is in the tail of its prior distribution determines the extent to which the target is in the tail of its posterior distribution.

6.2   Ecological Inference, Revisited

Recall from Chapter 2 that a simple form of the ecological inference problem arises in trying to infer a property of a bivariate distribution when the only available data pertain to the two corresponding univariate marginal distributions. This provided an accessible introductory problem with which to demonstrate some partially identified model fundamentals. In essence, marginals reveal something, but not everything, about joint distributions.

An important generalization of the ecological inference problem arises when we have data on marginal distributions for a number of study populations. For instance, there have been many epidemiologic studies considering per-country data on dietary consumption and disease incidence. These kinds of studies lead to claims such as Mediterranean diets are protective against cardiovascular disease. Recall from Example A in Chapter 2 that marginal distributions induce bounds on joint properties. Now suppose that an exposure-disease association measure, such as an odds-ratio, were constant across countries. The marginal data from a single country would then contribute a bound on this association. And intersecting the bounds contributed by numerous countries could then tighten inference, whilst still remaining in the domain of partial identification. The assumption of constant association across countries is too strong to be defensible in most situations, but this can be relaxed via a random effects model. That is, we can postulate the association to be similar across countries.

For some entry points to this literature, see Morgenstern (1995), Wakefield (2004), Wakefield (2008), and King (2013).

Example I: Gene-Environment Interaction and Disjoint Data Sources

Say that interest is focused on a binary genotype variable G, a binary environmental exposure variable X, and a binary outcome variable Y. More particularly, quantities describing the conditional distribution of $(Y|X,G)$ are to be inferred. For instance, say the inferential target is

$$\psi \quad = \quad Pr(Y=1|X=1,G=1) - Pr(Y=1|X=0,G=1), \quad (6.5)$$

interpreted as the risk difference with environmental exposure, amongst the genotype $G=1$ subpopulation.

If (X,Y,G) are jointly observable, then the task at hand, inferring (6.5), is straightforward. Our situation, however, is that information about the (Y,G) marginal distribution and information about the X distribution arise from disjoint sources. In this sense we do have an ecological inference problem, albeit a rather specialized one. In practice this situation could arise because the cost of per-person measurement of X is far greater than that of Y or G. So it may be attractive to capture (Y,G) for subjects in the current study, while relying on previous studies for information about X. Various versions of this problem, and further discussion on circumstances where it arises, can be found in Gustafson (2010), Gustafson and Burstyn (2011), Luo et al. (2013), and Gustafson (2014).

One version of this problem would be that two independent data samples are available: one in which (Y,G) are recorded and the other in which X is recorded. In terms of studying limiting posterior distributions then, we could investigate what happens when the sizes of both samples go to infinity. In fact, we simply take the X prevalence in the study population, $r = Pr(X=1)$, to be a known constant. Then we ask what happens to inference based on a single sample of (Y,G), in the limit of increasing sample size. This is mathematically equivalent to considering two independent samples of increasing size; however, the details are slightly easier to exposit.

To contrast how informative the data are against a backdrop of *a priori* assumptions, we consider what we can learn about ψ from the distribution of (Y,G) under three successively stronger assumptions.

Assumption A: No further assumptions, beyond r being known.

Assumption B: Assumption A, plus the further assumption that X and G are independent of one another in the source population. This is commonly referred to as the *gene-environment independence* (GEI) assumption.

Assumption C: Assumption B, plus the further assumption that genotype alone has no influence on disease risk in the absence of environmental exposure. Mathematically, this is expressed as

$$Pr(Y = 1 | G = 0, X = 0) \quad = \quad Pr(Y = 1 | G = 1, X = 0).$$

Qualitatively, this asserts that G has no "main effect," and if it does influence the outcome, this must be via an "interaction" with X. That is, G is known *a priori* to be only an *effect modifier*.

Before proceeding, we note that the GEI assumption is often biologically plausible, given the randomized manner in which genes are passed to offspring. Consequently, there is now a sizeable literature on exploiting the assumption for statistical gain. We have more to say on this below. The assumption that genotype is only an effect modifier is less generally applicable. For discussion on when this assumption is appropriate, see Burstyn et al. (2009) and Gustafson and Burstyn (2011).

Determining the Identification Interval

We start by working out the identification region for the target (6.5) and comparing it with the range of *a priori* plausible values, $\psi \in [-1, 1]$. It is convenient to do this first under Assumption B. From here, the analysis can be tweaked to deal with either the weaker Assumption A or the stronger Assumption C. As another convenience, rather than thinking of data in the form of bivariate observations of (Y, G), we think of $q = Pr(G = 1)$ being known, while data arise in the form of $(Y | G)$ observations, i.e., a first sample from $(Y | G = 0)$ and a second sample from $(Y | G = 1)$. Again for purposes of studying the large-sample limit, this makes no material difference.

Let μ_{xg} parameterize $(Y | X, G)$ according to $\mu_{xg} = Pr(Y = 1 | X = x, G = g)$. Then $\theta = (\mu_{00}, \mu_{01}, \mu_{10}, \mu_{11})$ is a scientific parameterization, with respect to which the target (6.5) is expressed as $\psi = \tilde{g}(\theta) = \mu_{11} - \mu_{01}$. However, the likelihood of the observable $(Y | G)$ data depends only on $\phi = (\phi_0, \phi_1)$, where

$$
\begin{aligned}
\phi_g \quad &= \quad Pr(Y = 1 | G = g) \\
&= \quad Pr(X = 0 | G = g) Pr(Y = 1 | X = 0, G = g) +
\end{aligned}
$$

$$Pr(X = 1|G = g)Pr(Y = 1|X = 1, G = g)$$
$$= \quad (1 - r)\mu_{0g} + r\mu_{1g}. \tag{6.6}$$

Note that here Assumption B has indeed been invoked, in order to obtain the last equality. If $\lambda = (\lambda_0, \lambda_1)$ is defined via $\lambda_g = \mu_{1g} - \mu_{0g}$, then $(\phi, \lambda) = h(\theta)$ is indeed a transparent reparameterization of θ. This is attested to by the explicit form of the inverse mapping $h^{-1}()$ as

$$\begin{pmatrix} \mu_{0g} \\ \mu_{1g} \end{pmatrix} = \begin{pmatrix} \phi_g - r\lambda_g \\ \phi_g + (1 - r)\lambda_g \end{pmatrix}, \tag{6.7}$$

for $g = 0, 1$.

Recalling that our interest parameter is $\psi = \lambda_1$, we can "read off" the identification interval from the $g = 1$ case of (6.7). That is, for fixed ϕ_1 the inverse mapping yields legitimate probabilities if and only if

$$\psi \quad \in \quad \left[-\min\left\{ \frac{1 - \phi_1}{r}, \frac{\phi_1}{1 - r} \right\}, \min\left\{ \frac{\phi_1}{r}, \frac{1 - \phi_1}{1 - r} \right\} \right]. \tag{6.8}$$

As a first comment, this identification interval is always *strictly* contained in the prior interval $\psi \in [-1, 1]$, except in the very special case that $\phi_1 = r = 0.5$. To confirm this, say $r \neq 0.5$. Then the left endpoint of (6.8) is strictly above -1 unless $\phi_1 = 1 - r$, in which case the right endpoint is strictly below 1. Similarly the right endpoint is strictly below 1 unless $\phi = r$, in which case the left endpoint is strictly above -1. Of course an obvious inferential limitation of (6.8) is that for every value of ϕ_1, the interval crosses zero. That is, an infinite amount of data plus a correct assertion of Assumption B can never reveal the *direction* of the effect of interest with complete certainty.

To adapt this analysis to Assumption A, let $\delta_g = Pr(X = 1|G = g)$, for $g = 0, 1$. Without the GEI assumption, we no longer have $\delta_0 = \delta_1 = r$. If δ_1 were known, then it could be substituted into (6.8) in place of r, and we would be done. All that is known about the (X, G) distribution, however, is $r = Pr(X = 1)$ and $q = Pr(G = 1)$. From the Fréchet bounds for $Pr(X = 1, G = 1)$ then, we know only that $\delta_1 \in [r_L, r_H]$, with $r_L = \max\{0, 1 - (1 - r)/q\}$ and $r_H = \min\{1, r/q\}$. Consequently, the identification interval is

$$\psi \quad \in \quad \left[-\min\left\{ 1, \frac{1 - \phi_1}{r_L}, \frac{\phi_1}{1 - r_H} \right\}, \min\left\{ 1, \frac{\phi_1}{r_L}, \frac{1 - \phi_1}{1 - r_H} \right\} \right]. \tag{6.9}$$

With a range of values (r_L, r_H) replacing r, it follows that (6.9) strictly contains (6.8). Or, put another way, correct invocation of the GEI assumption always reduces uncertainty about the target parameter. It is also easy to verify empirically that depending on ϕ, (6.9) can have zero, one, or two endpoints in common with the prior interval $[-1, 1]$. With only assumption A then, total futility can arise. At some points in the parameter space, an infinite amount of data would not rule out any *a priori* plausible values of the target.

Just as we can weaken Assumption B, we can also strengthen it, to Assumption C. To do so, we replace the scientific parameterization with $\theta = (\mu_0, \mu_{10}, \mu_{11})$, where $\mu_0 = Pr(Y = 1|X = 0, G = 0) = Pr(Y = 1|X = 0, G = 1) = Pr(Y = 1|X = 0)$, while, as before, $\mu_{1g} = Pr(Y = 1|X = 1, G = g)$, for $g = 0, 1$. In this case, (ϕ_0, ϕ_1, ψ) constitutes a transparent reparameterization, as per (6.6), but with μ_{0g} replaced by μ_0. As determined in Gustafson (2014), the inverse mapping for this case is

$$
\begin{pmatrix} \mu_0 \\ \mu_{10} \\ \mu_{11} \end{pmatrix} = r^{-1} \begin{pmatrix} 0 & r & -r^2 \\ 1 & -(1-r) & r(1-r) \\ 0 & r & r(1-r) \end{pmatrix} \begin{pmatrix} \phi_0 \\ \phi_1 \\ \psi \end{pmatrix}. \quad (6.10)
$$

From here, the requirement that μ_0 and μ_{11} be probabilities induces exactly the same restrictions as under Assumption B. But now the requirement that μ_{10} be a probability induces a further constraint on ψ, that depends on both ϕ_0 and ϕ_1. Assembling the pieces, we have the identification interval as

$$
\psi \in \left[- \min\left\{ \frac{1-\phi_1}{r}, \frac{\phi_1}{1-r}, \frac{\phi_0 - (1-r)\phi_1}{r(1-r)} \right\}, \right.
$$
$$
\left. \min\left\{ \frac{\phi_1}{r}, \frac{1-\phi_1}{1-r}, \frac{r+(1-r)\phi_1 - \phi_0}{r(1-r)} \right\} \right]. \quad (6.11)
$$

It is easy to check that the extra constraint may or may not be binding. That is, for some values of ϕ, (6.11) is strictly contained in (6.8), while for others the two intervals are identical. It is also easy to verify that the nature of the additional constraint precludes it from being binding at both ends of the interval. That is, (6.11) must have at least one endpoint in common with (6.8). Finally, and importantly, for some values of ϕ (6.11) excludes zero. At some points in the parameter space then, we will learn the effect direction with certainty, as the sample size grows.

Demonstration

To compare the information available when the various assumptions are imposed, we invoke Assumption C and generate 1000 sets of $(q, r, \mu_0, \mu_{10}, \mu_{11})$ values by simulating each of the five quantities independently from the Unif$(0, 1)$ distribution. For each set we then compute the three identification intervals, as per (6.9), (6.8) and (6.11) for Assumptions A, B and C, respectively.

We find that invoking Assumption A gives an identification interval that coincides with the prior interval of $(-1, 1)$ for 37.1% of the generated scenarios. With only Assumption A then, learning nothing from an infinite amount of data is a distinct possibility! For 26.0% of the generated scenarios, the identification interval has exactly one endpoint in common with the prior interval, i.e., the data rule out values at one end of the prior interval, but not the other. And, as must follow, for the remaining 36.9% of generated values, the identification interval is strictly contained in the prior interval. That is, via the data some progress is made in excluding values at both ends of the prior interval. As an aggregate measure of what is gained from the data plus Assumption A, the geometric mean of the ratio of the A interval length to the prior interval length is 0.759.

Turning to the B identification interval, we already know this is guaranteed to be strictly contained by the A identification interval, and therefore by the prior interval. The A and B interval lengths are compared in the left panel of Figure 6.5. As a measure of the typical reduction in length when imposing Assumption B rather than just Assumption A, the geometric mean of the ratio of interval lengths (B to A) is 0.734.

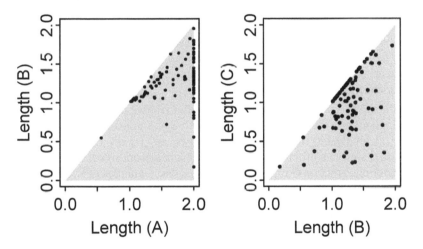

Figure 6.5 *Comparison of identification interval widths under various assumptions in Example I. For 1000 parameter values generated from a uniform distribution, the interval widths for Assumptions A and B (left panel) and Assumptions B and C (right panel) are compared.*

Moving to Assumption C, the B and C interval lengths are compared in the right panel of Figure 6.5. It transpires that for 41.3% of the scenarios, the B and C identification intervals are identical. Thus there is often "no return on investment" for correctly invoking the assumption that G can act only as an effect modifier for X. On the other hand, for 17.1% of scenarios, the Assumption C identification interval excludes zero. Thus in a minority of situations there is a good return, with the data able to conclusively determine the effect direction. The "typical return" is summarized by the geometric mean of the ratio of lengths (C to B) being 0.742.

In all, we tend to see about a 25% reduction in interval length each time we strengthen the assumption. Of course these geometric means of ratios can be combined multiplicatively. For instance, the geometric mean of the ratio of the length of the Assumption C identification interval to the length of the prior interval is $0.759 \times 0.736 \times 0.742 \approx 0.41$. This speaks to data collection being worthwhile when Assumption C is defensible, as we might typically reduce the range of plausible target values by more than a factor of two.

Determining the Limiting Posterior Distribution

In the case of Assumption C, we now consider the limiting posterior distribution on the target parameter. In fact, this is a situation where much of the action has already happened by the time we have determined the identification interval. Particularly, an obvious prior distribution to consider is a uniform distribution on $(\mu_0, \mu_{10}, \mu_{11})$. But, as is seen from (6.10), the map between θ and (ϕ_0, ϕ_1, ψ) is linear. Hence the prior distribution of (ϕ_0, ϕ_1, ψ) is also uniform, so that the LPD for ψ must be the uniform distribution over the identification interval (6.11). Properties of the LPD are then trivially inferred from properties of the identification interval.

As noted by Gustafson (2014), the situation is more complicated if different priors are specified for θ. Generally with a non-uniform prior for θ, the data speak loudly, i.e., distinct parameter values can give rise to the same identification interval but different limiting posterior distributions over this interval. In fact, for this problem Gustafson (2014) uses the techniques of Section 2.7 to understand the information flow, by comparing an ad-hoc distribution over the identification interval, the coarsened limiting posterior distribution (CLPD), and the actual limiting posterior distribution. The findings are generally similar to those for Example A in Section 2.7. Almost all of the benefit of Bayesian inference is available from the CLPD, though there is a demonstrably non-zero further benefit of the LPD compared to the CLPD. ∎

Aside: A Variety of Purposes for Genotype Independence Assumptions

It is interesting that independence assumptions concerning genotypes can be employed in rather different ways. The crux of the argument is that there is random assortment of alleles at the time of gamete formation, so that genetic variants can reasonably be assumed independent of various behavioral and environmental variables. However, one line of inquiry actually seeks to find genetic variants that are exceptions to this pattern. That is, variants which seem to influence behavior are sought. For example, variants have been found which are correlated with alcohol consumption, with milk consumption, and with leafy vegetable consumption. Linking back to Chapter 5, such a variant is a prime candidate to be an instrumental variable. For instance, to study an association between alcohol consumption as the exposure and a particular disease as the outcome, such a variant would be associated with the exposure, but plausibly independent of unobserved confounders of the exposure-disease relationship. And plausibly the variant would not have a direct effect on the outcome. Thus the conditions for being an instrumental variable would be satisfied. Colloquially, using a genetic variant as an instrumental variable has come to be known as using "Mendelian randomization." For entry points to this literature, see Smith and Ebrahim (2003), Smith and Ebrahim (2004), Sacerdote et al. (2007), and Lawlor et al. (2008).

On the other hand, sometimes for the exposure and disease at hand, a variant might plausibly interact with the exposure in its effect on outcome, whilst also plausibly being independent of this exposure. In this case, the phrasing "gene-environment independence" tends to be used, rather than Mendelian randomization. And, as we have seen in Example I, invoking the assumption can result in sharper inferences. Entry points to this literature include Umbach and Weinberg (1998), Chatterjee and Carroll (2005), Kraft et al. (2007), and Chen and Chen (2011). ★

Chapter 7

Further Topics

7.1 Computational Considerations

It is this author's contention that computation with partially identified models is a "bottleneck" issue. Throughout this monograph, we have relied on the concept that for the statistical model at hand we can identify a transparent parameterization. Unfortunately, though, statistical "real-life" is often messier than this.

To illustrate the computational bottleneck, we turn to the problem of unobserved confounding, and a family of statistical models that have received considerable recent attention in the literature (see, for instance, McCandless et al., 2007, 2008; Gustafson et al., 2010; McCandless et al., 2012). An archetype of these models can be expressed as follows. The goal is to investigate the conditional association between an outcome Y and a binary exposure X, given some covariates (C, U). The covariates are split according to C being observable and U being unobservable, presuming that C could contain one or more variables, while U is restricted to being a single variable.

For the case of a binary outcome, a logistic regression relationship for the outcome might be envisioned, say limited to main effects only, as per

$$\text{logit } Pr(Y = 1 | X, C, U) \quad = \quad \beta_0 + \beta_x X + \beta_c^T C + \alpha_u U. \qquad (7.1)$$

Here β_x would typically be the parameter of most inferential interest. Of course with U unobserved, (7.1) cannot be directly fitted to data. Rather, it is combined with a model for U. Presuming U is also binary, another logistic regression relationship can be employed, again with only main effect terms say:

$$\text{logit} Pr(U = 1 | X, C) = \alpha_0 + \alpha_x X + \alpha_c^T C. \qquad (7.2)$$

Taken together, (7.1) and (7.2) define a model for $(Y, U | X, C)$, and hence a model for $(Y | X, C)$, parameterized by $\theta = (\alpha, \beta)$.

The situation is nuanced depending on the number of components of C and their type (i.e., binary, continuous), but we lack a general strategy to reparameterize θ in a transparent way. Even in the special case that C is comprised of p binary covariates, the situation is unclear. In this special case, $\dim(\theta) = 2p + 5$, whereas the distribution of $(Y | X, C)$ is characterized by 2^{p+1} cell probabilities.

141

With $p \leq 2$, nonidentification is guaranteed, since there are more parameters than learnable cell probabilities. However, a malleable transparent parameterization in these situations seems elusive. When $p > 2$, there are fewer parameters than learnable cell probabilities, so that identification is not ruled out, but nor is it guaranteed. And identification would seem "unlikely" on intuitive grounds, since so little is assumed about how U relates to the observed variables. But again a mathematical route to shedding light on the situation seems elusive.

The crux of the situation is that we lack theoretical insight into even quite basic questions about what is going on. Most particularly, we cannot say anything about the limiting posterior marginal distribution of α compared to the prior marginal distribution of α. That is, we cannot confirm or refute the intuition that data carry little, if any, information about α. This is a pertinent issue in that related methodologies for unobserved confounding problems take this lack of information as a starting premise. Notably, "probabilistic bias analysis" and "Monte Carlo sensitivity analysis" have been proposed as methodologies to deal with unobserved confounding and other problems (see, for instance, Greenland, 2003, 2005; Lash et al., 2009). These procedures, while having a "veneer of Bayesianity," do compel the prior and "posterior-like" distributions of parameters connecting U to (Y,X,C) to be identical. Hence it would be nice to have a better understanding of how closely this property is mimicked by a fully Bayesian approach.

Given the lack of a theoretical insight into this, and other, partially identified models, we would like to fall back on computation of the posterior distribution for given datasets. Even this is problematic, however. Often Bayesian computation for models involving latent quantities is best tackled by going after the joint posterior distribution of parameters and latent variables. In the present context then, this would mean computing the joint posterior distribution of $(\alpha, \beta, u_{1:n})$ given the observed data $(y_{1:n}, x_{1:n}, c_{1:n})$. General experience with MCMC applied to this target distribution is not encouraging though. Very bad mixing is seen for off-the-shelf MCMC approaches, e.g., the algorithms "under the hood" if we use general-purpose Bayesian software such as Win-BUGS (Lunn et al., 2009). In the specific situation of the model arising from (7.1) and (7.2), McCandless et al. (2007) do give a specially tailored MCMC scheme that works tolerably with some datasets, though the performance tends to degrade as the sample size increases. And in variants of the problem, such as that described in Gustafson et al. (2010) where U and C are continuous, the approach targeting the joint distribution of parameters and latent variables seems to break down completely. Thus Gustafson et al. (2010) actually advocate applying MCMC to the joint posterior distribution of the parameters alone, even though the requisite likelihood evaluations require numerical quadrature, to remove the latent U. And to further complicate matters, very specialized proposal distributions must be devised, and the resulting algorithm is highly brittle. For instance, there is no obvious algorithmic tweak to move from continuous C to categorical C. So, in problems like these, trying to address subtle questions about information flow via empirical calculation is difficult.

Ideally we could focus attention on specifying the most realistic models and prior distributions for the problem at hand, with posterior computation "farmed out" to a black-box algorithm. At least we have some intuition about why this often does not work. A default MCMC strategy would work with the initial parameterization θ and attempt to update one component of θ at a time, with the other components remaining fixed. This, however, does not reflect the structure of a partially identified problem. *If* we could identify a transparent parameterization (ϕ, λ), then we could use "narrow" MCMC proposal distributions to update elements of ϕ, reflecting the impact of the data on narrowing the posterior distribution of ϕ. And by the same token, we could use "wide" proposals for λ, to reflect the lack of data influence for inference on these procedures. Or, even better, we could attempt a further reparameterization, to ensure a loose, rather than sticky, transparent reparameterization. Then the strategy of appropriately using wide and narrow proposal distributions is likely to be particularly effective. However, absent the ability to find a transparent reparameterization, these intuitions cannot be harnessed for computational gain. For situations where identification is known, or suspected, not to hold, fresh new ideas about posterior computation are sorely needed!

Several recent papers do make some small steps toward elucidating posterior distributions when identification is lacking but a transparent parameterization cannot be found. Gustafson (2009) gives an algorithm to determine the limiting posterior distribution when a transparent parameterization cannot be found, but a transparent "overparameterization" can be written down. That is, θ can be cleaved as $\theta = (\theta_a, \theta_b)$, the distribution of the data depends on θ only through $\phi = h(\theta)$, and the value of θ can be readily determined from (ϕ, θ_a), with $\dim(\phi) + \dim(\theta_a) > \dim(\theta)$. While this expands the collection of partially identified models for which we can study the limiting posterior distribution, it is far from a panacea. It does not help, for instance, with the unobserved confounding model described above.

Another recent paper pushing the envelope on Bayesian inference in the absence of identification is Jones et al. (2010). These authors connect classical results on identification with Bayesian inference. Particularly, they draw on much earlier work connecting identification with mathematical properties of the mapping from parameters to cell probabilities (Rothenberg, 1971; Goodman, 1974; Shapiro, 1986) . Jones et al. (2010) use symbolic algebra software to obtain a singular value decomposition of the Jacobian of this map, in turn shedding light on which parameters in the original parameterization, if any, are identified.

7.2   Study Design Considerations

As alluded to earlier, if we take partial identification seriously then we need a complete rethinking of issues of study design generally, and sample size determination specifically. Almost all the literature on sample size determination looks at situations where estimator uncertainty falls off like $n^{-1/2}$. This premise enables various formulations of finding the n which reduces the uncertainty to a desired level.

A variety of schemes for Bayesian sample size determination have been put forth in the literature. As reviewed by M'Lan et al. (2006), for instance, criteria can be based on either average credible interval length or average credible interval coverage. Recall that in Chapter 2 we used $H_\pi^{(\alpha)}(\psi^*|d_n)$ to denote the highest posterior density set with posterior probability content $1 - \alpha$ for target ψ, having observed data d_n. Presuming this set is in fact an interval, we will now use $\|H_\pi^{(\alpha)}(\psi^*|d_n)\|$ to denote the interval length. We also introduce a related notation that $\tilde{H}_\pi^{(l)}(\psi^*|d_n)$ is the HPD credible interval of length l for the target. Thus $\tilde{H}_\pi^{(l)}(\psi^*|d_n) = H_\pi^{(\alpha)}(\psi^*|d_n)$ if and only if $\|H_\pi^{(\alpha)}(\psi^*|d_n)\| = l$.

Using these notations, an *average length criterion* would be based on specifying a desired α and l, and then selecting that smallest sample size n for which

$$E\left\{\|H_\pi^{(\alpha)}(\psi^\star|d_n^\star)\|\right\} \;\geq\; l. \tag{7.3}$$

That is, n is chosen so that the average length of the $(1 - \alpha)$ credible interval is as short as desired, where the average is with respect to the marginal distribution of the data. Alternately, for a specified α and l one could select the smallest n satisfying

$$E\,Pr\left\{\psi^\star \in \tilde{H}^{(l)}(\psi^\star|d_n^\star)|d_n^\star\right\} \;\geq\; 1 - \alpha. \tag{7.4}$$

This constitutes an *average coverage criterion*, insisting that the average posterior probability content of the credible interval of specified length be as high as desired. Again here the average is with respect to the marginal distribution of the data.

An important point about either (7.3) or (7.4) is that the specified prior distribution plays two roles. It is used in the determination of the posterior distribution for a given dataset, and it also induces the marginal distribution of the data used to average either the interval length or the interval coverage. In Chapter 1 we referred to the former role as that of the "investigator's prior," and the latter as that of "Nature's parameter-generating distribution," though the respective phrases "analysis prior" and "design prior" could also be applied. A key emphasis in Wang and Gelfand (2002) is that for purposes of sample size determination one might well wish to make the design prior differ from the analysis prior. Particularly, one may not wish to think subjectively in terms of doing the analysis, so that a diffuse analysis prior is employed. But one may be comfortable with fairly sharp *a priori* judgments feeding into the design prior. In fact, non-Bayesian approaches to sample size determination often require *very* sharp prior judgments about the parameter values under which calculations will be carried out, particularly when hypothesis testing is the goal. So the Bayesian approach with a design prior that averages over a range of plausible scenarios can in fact be more flexible than a frequentist approach that involves simply "plugging in" a single scenario.

Criteria such as (7.3) and (7.4) are *stated* in a manner which is blind to whether or not the target parameter is identified. It is important to note, however, that for a given partially identified model and target, and given choice of (α, l), it may not be possible to satisfy (7.3) and/or (7.4) at any n. That is, the LPD on the target may be too wide, in aggregated terms across the parameter space.

The main context in which sample size determination for partially identified models has arisen in the literature is that of a binary trait subject to misclassification (Rahme et al., 2000; Dendukuri et al., 2004; Stamey et al., 2005; Dendukuri et al., 2010; Joseph and Bélisle, 2013). Specifically, Rahme et al. (2000) consider a single surrogate for the trait of interest, measured in a single population. This is then extended to two conditionally independent nondifferential surrogates realized in a single population by Dendukuri et al. (2004). In both cases, it is explicitly acknowledged that for a given l and α it may not be possible to attain the desired guarantee at any sample size. Stamey et al. (2005) consider two populations with different prevalences of the trait of interest, with either one surrogate or two conditionally independent surrogates, and with or without the nondifferentiality assumption that the surrogates are conditionally independent of the population indicator given the true trait value. These authors also emphasize the qualitative difference between identified and nonidentified settings. In a different vein, Dendukuri et al. (2010) consider the single-population case, and examine the reduction in sample size needed if three conditionally independent surrogates are available, rather than just two. In some of their settings the reduction is very dramatic, precisely because the three-surrogate model is identified while the two-surrogate version is not.

To look in more detail at a situation relating to one of our examples, Joseph and Bélisle (2013) consider sample size determination in the same setting as our Example C from Chapter 3. Recall that this involves case-control analysis, with the binary exposure variable subject to misclassification. Joseph and Bélisle (2013) consider both nondifferential misclassification (as per Example C) and differential misclassification. In the former situation, they examine an array of settings involving different prior distributions on the four parameters and different target interval lengths (with $\alpha = 0.05$ throughout). Many of these settings are such that neither (7.3) nor (7.4) can be satisfied. That is, the desired length cannot be achieved because too much of the prior uncertainty about the misclassification parameters propagates through to the posterior distribution of the target.

The approach described above is a variant on the usual scheme for sample size determination. It involves inputting a desired narrowness of inference, and then calculating a sample size which gives some form of promise about meeting this desire. An entirely different approach was pursued in Gustafson (2006), with an emphasis on quantifying when "diminishing returns" kick in. As has been emphasized repeatedly in this book, a hallmark of partial identification is a relatively small sample size yielding a posterior distribution almost as narrow as what would be obtained from having infinite data. The idea in Gustafson (2006) is to quantify, in advance of data collection, a sample size beyond which further data collection constitutes a squandering of resources.

To explain, we have already seen in Chapter 2 that a transparent parameterization (ϕ, λ) presents a decomposition of the posterior variance on the target parameter $\psi = g(\phi, \lambda)$:

$$
\begin{aligned}
\mathrm{Var}_\pi\{\psi^*|d_n\} &= E_\pi[\mathrm{Var}_\pi\{g(\phi^\star,\lambda^\star)|\phi^\star,d_n\}|d_n] + \\
&\quad \mathrm{Var}_\pi[E_\pi\{g(\phi^\star,\lambda^\star)|\phi^\star\}|d_n] \\
&= E_\pi[E_\pi\{(g(\phi^\star,\lambda^\star)-g_\pi(\phi^\star))^2|\phi^\star,d_n\}|d_n] + \\
&\quad \mathrm{Var}_\pi[g_\pi(\phi^\star)|d_n] \\
&= E_\pi[\{g_\pi(\phi^\star)-g(\phi^\star,\lambda^\star)\}^2|d_n]+\mathrm{Var}_\pi\{g_\pi(\phi^\star)|d_n\}.
\end{aligned}
$$

From here we take expectation with respect to the marginal distribution of the data, to characterize the typical uncertainty across repeated *joint* sampling of $(\theta^\star, d_n^\star)$, thereby obtaining the *expected posterior variance* (EPV) of the target parameter:

$$
\begin{aligned}
EPV &= E_\pi[\mathrm{Var}_\pi\{\psi^*|d_n^\star\}] \\
&= E_\pi[\{g_\pi(\phi^\star)-g(\phi^\star,\lambda^\star)\}^2]+E_\pi[\mathrm{Var}_\pi\{g_\pi(\phi^\star)|d_n^\star\}]. \quad (7.5)
\end{aligned}
$$

Recall that $g_\pi(\phi) - g(\phi, \lambda)$ is the difference between the large-sample limit of the posterior mean for the target parameter and the target itself. In the above decomposition of *EPV* then, the first term can be regarded as the *average squared asymptotic bias* (ASAB), where the average is taken with respect to the prior distribution. Of course this term does not depend on the sample size, whereas the second term, the expected posterior variance of $g_\pi(\phi) = \int g(\phi, \lambda)\pi(\lambda|\phi)d\lambda$, falls off in proportion to n. So we can quantify the "march of knowledge," in terms of the EPV going from the prior variance of $g(\phi, \lambda)$ before any data is collected down to the *ASAB* in the limit of an infinite amount of data.

Toward operationalizing this, let

$$
v = E_\pi\{g_\pi'(\phi^\star)^T I(\phi^\star)^{-1}g_\pi'(\phi^\star)\}, \quad (7.6)
$$

where $I(\phi)$ is the Fisher information matrix based on a single observation from the identified model induced by the original model, i.e., an observation from $\pi(d_1|\phi)$. So approximately we have $E_\pi[\text{Var}_\pi\{g_\pi(\phi)|d_n^\star\}] \approx n^{-1}v$. In fact, a slightly more refined and useful approximation for present purposes is

$$E_\pi[\text{Var}_\pi\{g_\pi(\phi^\star)|d_n^\star\}] \approx \frac{1}{\text{Var}_\pi\{g_\pi(\phi^\star)\}+nv^{-1}}. \tag{7.7}$$

This mimics the additive property of prior and data precisions which is exact in models based on normal distributions and approximately correct otherwise. Upon noting that $\text{Var}_\pi\{g_\pi(\phi^\star)\} = \text{Var}_\pi\{g(\phi^\star,\lambda^\star)\} - ASAB$, we can combine (7.5) and (7.7) to approximate the expected posterior variance as

$$EPV = ASAB + \frac{1}{[\text{Var}_\pi\{\psi^\star\} - ASAB]^{-1}+nv^{-1}}. \tag{7.8}$$

Thus for a given partially identified model we can compute the prior variance of the target parameter, and the $ASAB$ and v terms. Via (7.8) then, this completely characterizes the reduction in expected posterior variance seen as the sample size increases.

An interesting feature of (7.8) is the contrast it presents between the partially identified and identified cases. As written, it applies to a partially identified model with target $g(\phi,\lambda)$. We can also consider what happens if we apply (7.8) when we think of $g_\pi(\phi)$ as the target, which puts us in the identified model realm. By changing the target, $ASAB$ is reduced to zero. Interestingly, however, $\text{Var}_\pi(\psi) - ASAB$ remains unchanged, as does v. Thus if we think of the EPV curve as a function of n, the impact of changing from the nonidentified target to the identified target is to shift the curve lower by $ASAB$ units.

Example J: Prevalence Estimation from Misclassified Data

Say that interest lies in estimating $r = E(Y = 1)$, the population prevalence of a binary trait Y. However, we observe independent and identically distributed realizations of a surrogate Y^* rather than Y, where the surrogate has perfect specificity but imperfect sensitivity. This could arise, for instance, in the context of a survey questionnaire, should there be a stigma attached with admitting to the $Y = 1$ status.

Let $\gamma = Pr(Y^* = 1|Y = 1)$ be the surrogate's sensitivity, and say the available prior knowledge involves a lower bound b for γ. More particularly, say the prior distribution $\gamma \sim \text{Unif}(b,1)$ is specified. As well, r and γ are taken as *a priori* independent, with $r \sim \text{Unif}(0,1)$.

Let $\phi = Pr(Y^* = 1) = r\gamma$ and let $\lambda = \gamma$. Immediately we see that (ϕ,λ) constitutes a transparent parameterization, since $Y^* \sim \text{Bernoulli}(\phi)$. Moreover, the target parameter is expressed as $r = g(\phi, \lambda) = \phi/\lambda$, while

$$\pi(\lambda|\phi) \quad \propto \quad \frac{1}{\lambda} I\{\max(b, \phi) < \lambda < 1\} \tag{7.9}$$

characterizes the limiting posterior distribution.

For what follows, it is useful to note that (7.9) implies

$$E\left(\frac{1}{\lambda^\star}\bigg|\phi\right) \quad = \quad \frac{1/\max(b,\phi) - 1}{-\log\max(b,\phi)},$$

and

$$\mathrm{Var}\left(\frac{1}{\lambda^\star}\bigg|\phi\right) \quad = \quad \frac{(1/2)(1/\max(b,\phi)^2 - 1)}{-\log\max(b,\phi)}.$$

To compute the requisite characteristics for this model, note that $\mathrm{Var}_\pi(\psi^\star) = \mathrm{Var}_\pi(r^\star) = 1/12$. Also,

$$
\begin{aligned}
ASAB \quad &= \quad E_\pi[\mathrm{Var}_\pi\{g(\phi^\star, \lambda^\star)|\phi^\star\}] \\
&= \quad E_\pi[\mathrm{Var}_\pi\{\phi^\star/\lambda^\star|\phi^\star\}] \\
&= \quad E_\pi\left[(\phi^\star)^2 \mathrm{Var}\{1/\lambda^\star|\phi^\star\}\right] \\
&= \quad E_\pi\left\{\frac{(\phi^\star)^2(1/\max(b,\phi^\star)^2 - 1)}{2(-\log\max(b,\phi^\star))}\right\},
\end{aligned}
$$

which can be simply computed via a Monte Carlo sample of $\phi^\star$ realizations drawn from the prior distribution. Similarly, (7.6) simplifies to

$$v \quad = \quad E_\pi\left[\phi^\star(1 - \phi^\star)\{g'_\pi(\phi^\star)\}^2\right],$$

which can also be evaluated as Monte Carlo average. To do so, note that

$$
\begin{aligned}
g_\pi(\phi) \quad &= \quad E(\phi^\star/\lambda^\star|\phi^\star = \phi) \\
&= \quad \phi(1/c(\phi) - 1)(-\log c(\phi))^{-1},
\end{aligned}
$$

where $c(\phi) = \max(b, \phi)$. Thus we can directly differentiate to get an expression for $g'_\pi(\phi)$, which in turn will involve $c'(\phi) = I\{\phi > b\}$. Using a Monte Carlo sample of size $10,000$, we obtain $ASAB = 0.002681$ (Monte Carlo SE $= 0.000022$) and $v = 0.2321$ (Monte Carlo SE $= 0.0013$). The resulting evolution of the expected posterior variance appears in Figure 7.1. Note this is given in terms of the square-root of EPV, i.e., the *root expected posterior variance*, $REPV = EPV^{1/2}$. The figure contrasts how $REPV$ falls off with sample size when estimating the actual target $\psi = r$ with the situation for estimating the identified quantity $\psi = g_\pi(\phi)$. Of course $REPV$ will asymptote to $ASAB^{1/2}$ in the former case and to zero in the latter case. ∎

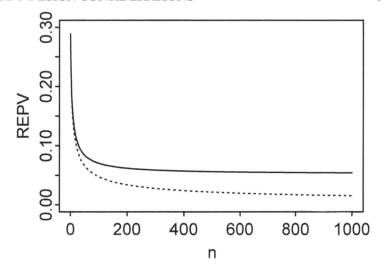

Figure 7.1 *Root expected posterior variance (REPV) in Example J, as a function of sample size. The solid curve arises from* $(a,b,v) = (0.002681, 0.083, 0.2321)$. *The dotted curve corresponds to taking* $g_\pi(\phi)$, *rather than* $g(\phi, \lambda)$, *as the target of inference.*

When is Further Data Collection not Worthwhile?

We can use (7.8) to quantify the sample size beyond which further data collection is "not worth it," as there is little scope for further reduction in EPV even if data collection were continued indefinitely. Let (a, s, v, c) be the characteristics of the study to be carried out, where a is the *ASAB* as defined above, $s = \text{Var}_\pi\{g(\phi^*, \lambda^*)\}$ is the prior variance of the target parameter, and v is as per (7.6), so that (a, s, v) completely characterize the evolution of the expected posterior variance with sample size according to (7.8). The further characteristic c is the "overhead cost" of the study, expressed in units of per-subject sampling cost. That is, the total cost of mounting the study, including the recruitment of n subjects, is proportional to $c + n$.

The other ingredient needed is a function $h()$ so that we measure the value of a study in the scale of the reduction in $h(EPV)$ rather than reduction in *EPV* itself. Gustafson (2006) provides arguments as to why $h(x) = p^{-1}x^p$, for $p \in (-1, 1)$, constitute sensible choices. Here $h(x) = \log x$ for $p = 0$, and in fact we use this particular choice of $h()$ in what follows.

Conceptually now, say a research team leader with fixed resources has to choose between doing many studies of different phenomena, each with quite a small sample size, or doing a few studies of different phenomena, each with a much larger sample size. And to keep things simple, say that for each phenomenon the same characteristics (a, s, v, c) apply. If the leader's global budget equates to the cost of sampling N subjects, then, should he choose to study k phenomena, the sample size for each study will necessarily be $N/k - c$. And the resulting aggregate reduction in $h(EPV)$ will be

$$\Delta_k = k\left[h(s) - h(a + \{(s-a)^{-1} + (k^{-1}N - c)v^{-1}\}^{-1})\right]. \quad (7.10)$$

Under this framework then, the number of studies k should simply be chosen to maximize (7.10). In turn, the optimal value of k leads to an optimal value of n, according to $n = N/k - c$. This framework then quantifies the notion that enlarging the sample size for a study may be suboptimal if the EPV is only slightly reduced, since these resources could be better used to commence a new study of a different phenomenon.

Gustafson (2006) shows that the solution to the above optimization problem can be cast in a slightly different form. Let $\text{val}(z)$ be the reduction in EPV attained by "spending" z study-subjects worth of resources on a single study. So

$$\text{val}(z) = \begin{cases} 0, & \text{if } z \le c, \\ h(s) - h(a + \{(s-a)^{-1} + (z-c)v^{-1}\}^{-1}), & \text{if } z > c. \end{cases}$$

Then the solution to the optimization problem can be cast as the value of z for which $\text{val}'(z) = \text{val}(z)/z$. This provides an intuitive interpretation that we should "keep going" (i.e., keep accruing subjects to the study) so long as the rate $\text{val}'(z)$ at which we are reducing $h(EPV)$ does not fall below the per-unit cost of the reduction attained thus far, $\text{val}(z)/z$. Graphically, the solution is seen as the value of z at which the $\text{val}()$ curve is tangent to a line through the origin.

Example J, Continued

Recall that values of (a, s, v) for this example are given above. Consider $h(x) = \log x$ (i.e., $p = 0$), and say $c = 250$, i.e., the overhead cost of a study equates with the cost of sampling 250 subjects. The value curve appears in the upper-left panel of Figure 7.2. The tangent line through the origin is also marked, revealing the optimal sample size (optimal cost minus initial cost c) of $n = 65$. The upper-right panel of Figure 7.2 repeats the analysis, but for the identified target quantity $g_\pi(\phi)$. So c and v remain unchanged, but (a, b) are replaced with $(0, b - a)$. We see that changing the target changes the geometry of the value curve, and now the optimal sample size is $n = 95$.

In the lower panels of Figure 7.2 this analysis is repeated, but now using $h(x) = -2/x^{1/2}$, i.e., $p = -0.5$. This yields a more marked contrast between the nonidentified and identified cases, with an optimal sample size of $n = 102$ for estimating $g(\phi, \lambda)$ compared to an optimal sample size of $n = 304$ for estimating $g_\pi(\phi)$. ■

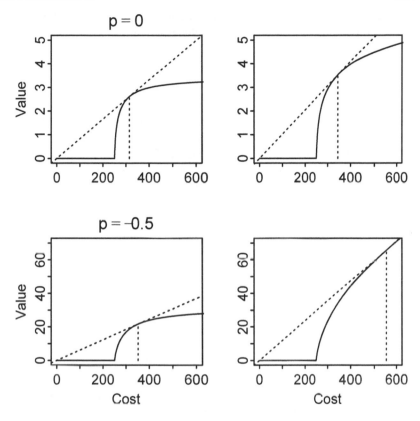

Figure 7.2 *Value versus cost in Example J, when the overhead cost corresponds to the cost of sampling c = 250 subjects. The left-hand panels correspond to the actual target of inference, with $(a,b,v) = (0.002681, 0.083, 0.2321)$. The right-hand panels correspond to taking $g_\pi(\phi)$ as the target of inference, i.e., (a,b) are replaced with $(\tilde{a},\tilde{b}) = (0,b-a)$. The upper panels use the logarithmic value function ($p = 0$), while the lower panels use $p = -0.5$. In each case the geometric interpretation of the optimal cost is indicated, corresponding to optimal sample sizes of $n = 65$ (partially identified target) and $n = 95$ (fully identified target) when $p = 0$, and $n = 102$ and $n = 304$ when $p = -0.5$.*

7.3   Applications

This book has been about the concepts and the mathematics of Bayesian inference in partially identified models. We have made extensive use of theoretical arguments and simulated data, in order to (i), compare inferences to "the truth," and (ii), see how evidence accumulates as data accumulate. Of course this is very important for our conceptual understanding of what is and is not possible. Ultimately, though, we want our conceptual understanding to inform the anal-

ysis of real data. Indeed, it should be stressed that the literature on Bayesian
inference in partially identified contexts includes a number of real-data examples. We mention some of these here, to impart some flavor of how partially
identified models can deal with limited data in the "trenches" of scientific research.

- Gustafson et al. (2001) consider data from a case-control study on a possible association between a genetic alteration and the development of head
  or neck cancer, in a population with premalignant oral lesions (Rosin et al.,
  2000). The alteration was detected in 32 of 87 controls, and in 28 of 29
  cases. The model studied in Example C is applied to these data, using prior
  distributions arising from discussions with subject-area experts. The specificity of the genetic test to detect the alteration is thought to be very high,
  i.e., false positives are unlikely. Thus a beta prior distribution with mode
  at 1 and 90% probability above 0.95 is assigned to the specificity. There is
  less confidence in the test's sensitivity, however, so a prior with mode at 0.9
  and 90% probability above 0.8 is used for this quantity. The resulting posterior distribution on the exposure-disease log odds-ratio (LOR) is wider than
  that obtained by pretending that the genetic test is perfect, with the added
  width manifested in the right tail rather than the left. For either analysis the
  distribution puts effectively all its mass above zero, so the evidence for a
  positive association is incontrovertible. A third analysis "plugs in" the prior
  modes of 0.9 for sensitivity and 1.0 for specificity, as if these were known
  values. For these data, this gives essentially the same posterior distribution
  for LOR as we get from acknowledging the uncertainty about sensitivity
  and specificity. One might then suggest that there is no point in using the
  partially identified model. However, we know generally, and with Example C particularly, that the situation is more nuanced than this. With some
  datasets we will see a qualitatively different answer upon acknowledging
  more uncertainty, and with others we will not. And importantly, of course,
  until we actually fit the partially identified model, we will not know which
  situation applies.

- Gustafson (2005a) considers data on systolic blood pressure and heart rate
  from the HARVEST study (Palatini et al., 1993), as described and reported
  by Schork and Remington (2000). For the $n = 311$ study subjects, let X^*
  and Y be suitably transformed versions of the measured systolic blood pressure and the measured heart rate. Given concern that X^*, as arises from a
  single measurement, can vary considerably around a "long-run average"
  blood pressure X, Gustafson (2005a) fits two versions of the following
  model:

$$
\begin{aligned}
X^*|Y,X &\sim N(X, r\lambda^2) \\
Y|X &\sim N(\beta_0 + \beta_1 X, \sigma^2) \\
X &\sim N(\mu, \lambda^2).
\end{aligned}
\tag{7.11}
$$

Note here particularly that r governs the quality of the blood-pressure measurement, in the relative sense of the ratio of measurement error variance to across-population variance in actual blood pressure. The model induces a bivariate normal distribution for the observables (X^*, Y), suggesting that five parameters could be consistently estimated. Commensurate with this, one version of the model involves taking r to be known, in which case identification results. Conversely, a version with an informative prior distribution for r, quantifying the notion that r is approximately known, is partially identified. For the HARVEST data, Gustafson (2005a) shows the wider posterior on the interest parameter β_1 that arises from treating r as approximately known, rather than exactly known. He also notes that replacing the linear relationship in (7.11) with a quadratic relationship renders the model identified, even if r is unknown. However, fitting the quadratic model rather than the linear model does *not* sharpen inference on β_1 for the HARVEST data. For these data there is no strong evidence that the relationship is indeed quadratic. Hence the observation that the quadratic model yields identification is of theoretical curiosity, but not of practical benefit.

- Gustafson (2007) takes up data from the Framingham heart study, doing an analysis relating to that reported in Carroll et al. (2006) [Sec. 6.5]. Here X is a transformed version of "long-run" systolic blood pressure at the time of a particular study visit, while Y is a binary indicator of the development of coronary heart disease over a long follow-up period. The goal is to infer the conditional association between X and Y, given some observable confounding variables Z.

Measurement error is a concern, in that X is latent, with a noisy surrogate X^* observed instead, based on measured blood pressure at the study visit. Also available is S, the surrogate measured at an *earlier* study visit. A seemingly sensible way to assemble these puzzle pieces is via the following model:

$$X^*|Y,X,S,Z \sim N(X, \tau^2),$$
$$\text{logit } Pr(Y=1|X,S,Z) = \beta_0 + \beta_x X + \beta_s S + \beta_z^T Z,$$
$$X|S,Z \sim N(\alpha_0 + \alpha_s S + \alpha_z^T Z, \lambda^2),$$

which in turn describes the observable distribution of $(X^*, Y|S, Z)$. There is a strong connection between this model to deal with measurement error in X and the Example G model from Section 5.3, which used an approximate instrumental variable to deal with unobserved confounding. In the present instance, supposing that S is an exact instrumental variable corresponds to supposing that $\beta_s = 0$, while supposing that S is an approximate instrumental variable corresponds to assigning a prior to β_s with most of its mass very close to zero.

In the closely related model in which Y is continuous and the logistic regression model for $(Y|X,S,Z)$ is replaced with a normal linear regression model, Gustafson (2007) shows that the approximate IV assumption induces partial identification, whereas the exact IV assumption induces full identification. In the case of binary Y, however, Gustafson (2007) shows that full identification arises *without* supposing that $\beta_2 = 0$. This transpires to be a theoretical rather than practical gain though. For the Framingham study data, the posterior marginal distribution on β_s is seen to be virtually identical to the prior marginal distribution. So the user must commit to a prior judgment limiting the likely extent to which S could have a direct influence on the outcome Y, for the data will remain largely silent on this issue. More positively for practical purposes, however, with the prior mean of β_s fixed at zero, increasing the prior standard deviation from zero induces only a modest widening of the marginal posterior distribution on the interest parameter β_x. At least for these data then, the assumption that S is exactly an instrumental variable can be weakened, without a large increase in uncertainty about the target parameter.

- Gustafson et al. (2010) consider data on female bone mineral density from a twin study conducted by Hopper and Seeman (1994), as also considered by Rosner (2000). Here Y is the within-pair difference in bone density at the femoral neck, while X is the within-pair difference in height. The goal is to consider the (X, Y) association adjusted for a vector of covariates Z. There is concern, however, about how well these covariates are measured. Thus the model postulates that the observed covariate vector Z^* constitutes a noisy surrogate for the actual covariate vector Z. Moreover, there is concern that the available covariates may not completely control for confounding, so the existence of a further unmeasured confounder U is postulated. Thus models for $(Z|X)$, $(U|Z,X)$, $(Y|U,Z,X)$, and $(Z^*|Y,U,Z,X)$ are combined, resulting in a model for the observable distribution of $(Z^*,Y|X)$. A supposition that the unobservable covariate U is exchangeable with the hard-to-measure covariates Z is used to reduce the model complexity, i.e., to limit the number of unknown parameters.

  Applying this model to the data at hand, the posterior mean for the X coefficient in the $(Y|U,X,Z)$ relationship is virtually the same as the naïve estimate obtained directly from the $(Y|X,Z^*)$ regression. However, the posterior standard deviation in the former case is nearly double that of the latter. This is the price paid for admitting that the available covariates Z may not completely control for confounding. Moreover, for these data the increase in posterior standard deviation results in a 95% credible interval crossing zero, whereas the naïve analysis produces an interval excluding zero. Thus we have a situation of "significance lost."

- Gustafson and Greenland (2009), following upon work of Steenland and Greenland (2004), reexamine data on lung cancer deaths in an occupational cohort of workers with high silica exposures. In particular, the observed number of deaths Y is compared to the expected number of deaths c, where c is determined from lung-cancer mortality rates in the general population, accounting for age, race, sex and calendar time of the cohort. A central challenge is lack of data on smoking behavior for cohort members, prompting the model

$$Y \sim \text{Poisson} \left[\exp \left\{ \log c + \beta_1 + \log(p_1 + p_2 e^{\beta_2} + p_3 e^{\beta_3}) - \right. \right.$$
$$\left. \left. \log(q_1 + q_2 e^{\beta_2} + q_3 e^{\beta_3}) \right\} \right].$$

Here β_1 is the log relative risk of lung cancer death for silica exposure versus no exposure, while β_2 and β_3 are log relative risks that compare current smokers to never smokers and former smokers to never smokers, respectively. The proportions $p = (p_1, p_2, p_3)$, which sum to one, give the distribution of smoking behavior (never, current, former) across this occupational cohort. Similarly, $q = (q_1, q_2, q_3)$ gives the distribution of smoking behavior across the general population. With β, p and q being unknown parameters, this model is clearly very far from identified. Identification results from the strong assumption that $p = q$, so that β_1 is the only parameter influencing Y, i.e., under this assumption smoking no longer confounds the association of interest. It turns out that previous studies and data sources yield defensible and quite informative prior distributions for β_2, β_3, p and q, with this prior information reflecting more smoking in the occupational cohort than in the general population. Using this prior information yields $(1.12, 1.73)$ as a 95% credible interval for $\exp(\beta_1)$, compared to $(1.31, 1.91)$ arising from the assumption that there is no confounding due to smoking.

Gustafson and Greenland (2009) also use this example to showcase an application of the basic calibration property of Bayesian interval estimation emphasized in Sections 1.3 and 2.6. They report Bayesian coverage for various choices of "Nature's parameter-generating distribution," with the investigator's prior fixed as per the reported main analysis. For these data and this investigator's prior, there is a considerable degree of robustness exhibited. Taking Nature's parameter-generating distribution to be various tweaked versions of the investigator's prior does not change the Bayesian coverage very much from the nominal level.

- Gustafson (2009) takes up data from Kosinski and Flanders (1999), which involve two imperfect measurements of a binary trait, in multiple populations. A version of the model from Example E (Section 4.2) is applied. The unobservable trait of interest X is whether a subject's coronary artery disease is hemodynamically obstructive or not, with the surrogates X_1^* and X_2^* being based on an exercise stress test and single-photon emission computed tomography, respectively. Data from three populations are considered: females, males weighing less than 90 kg, and males weighing 90 kg or more. As in Example E, a prior which modestly downweights stronger conditional association of $(X_1^*, X_2^*|X)$ is used. The data, on $n = 307$ subjects in total, turn out to be only moderately informative concerning the X prevalence in the three populations and the characteristics of the two surrogates. Gustafson (2009) also focuses on sample size progression with these data, showing that in fact a reduction of sample size by a factor of four does not greatly increase posterior uncertainty. He also considers the large-sample limit of the posterior with the parameters fixed at estimated values. In this limit the posterior marginal distributions are not much more concentrated than those seen with the actual data.

Chapter 8

Concluding Thoughts

8.1 What Have Others Said?

It is interesting to look at some of the opinions expressed by those who have
grappled with Bayesian inference in partially identified contexts, both histor-
ically and recently. One oft-quoted sentiment comes from Lindley (1972, p.
46). In the context of discussing a particular statistical model, he remarks, in a
footnote:

> In passing it might be noted that unidentifiability causes no real diffi-
> culties in the Bayesian approach. If the likelihood does not involve a
> particular parameter, θ_1 say, when written in the natural form, then the
> conditional distribution of θ_1, given the remaining parameters, will be
> the same before and after the data. This will not typically be true of
> the marginal distribution of θ_1 because of the changes in assessment of
> the other parameters caused by the data, though if θ_1 is independent of
> them, it will be. For example, unidentifiable (or unestimable) parame-
> ters in linear least squares theory are like θ_1, and do not appear in the
> likelihood. Notice, however, that with certain types of prior distribution
> having strong association between θ_1 and the other parameters, data not
> involving θ_1 can provide a lot of information about it. Effectively this is
> what happens in the case under discussion.

The mantra of "no real difficulties," in that a proper prior distribution will
always lead to a proper posterior distribution no matter what, has endured. For
instance, Aldrich (2002) cites Lindley's remark, referring to it as a "talisman"
for Bayesian econometrics. Poirier (1998, p. 483) also takes Lindley's remark
as a starting point, before going on to say that:

> The "solution" to an identification problem is also in common agree-
> ment: more information is required, and this usually means non-
> data-based information. Here, however, paths begin to diverge. Non-
> Bayesians introduce dogmatic restrictions on the unknown parameters
> until identification is achieved. Bayesians may do so as well, but they
> also have the option of introducing nondogmatic information via a prior
> distribution. Lindley's quote ... refers to the fact that a Bayesian analysis

of a nonidentified model is always possible if a proper prior on all the parameters is specified.

Poirier (1998) goes on to present a number of examples for which, in his words, "prior dependence between identified and nonidentified parameters arises naturally." Linking back to our terminology, he is emphasizing that indirect learning about target parameters is a fundamental concept pertaining to partial identification.

In a similar spirit to Lindley, Neath and Samaniego (1997, p. 226) also reinforce the idea that you can turn the Bayesian crank, no matter what:

> In contrast to the classical approach, Bayesian methods can provide point estimates of a nonidentifiable parameter that are unambiguous and unique (relative to a given prior). The mechanics of Bayesian inference will pose the usual challenges—the appropriate quantification of the prior distribution and the derivation of the posterior distribution— but these challenges do not become impenetrable by virtue of the nonidentifiability of the parameter. Bayesian analysis in these problems thus constitutes a rational method for producing a point estimate, a method that has no natural classical counterpart.

Expounding upon the choice between Bayesian and frequentist approaches, several authors emphasize what we referred to in Chapter 3 as the contrast between working with a nonidentified model or forcing identification via overly strong assumptions. For instance, in the context of a diagnostic test without any gold-standard reference, Joseph et al. (1995, p. 264) write:

> The basic idea behind the Bayesian approach presented here is to eliminate the need for these constraints by first constructing a prior distribution over all unknown quantities. The data, through the likelihood function, are then combined with the prior distribution to derive posterior distributions using Bayes' theorem. This allows simultaneous inferences to be made on all parameters. The posterior distributions contain updated beliefs about the values of the model parameters, after taking into account the information provided by the data. This procedure can be viewed as a generalization of the frequentist approach, since the latter's constrained parameters can be considered to have degenerate marginal prior distributions with probability mass equal to one on their constrained values, while the lack of prior information assumed for the unconstrained parameters can be represented by a uniform or other noninformative prior distribution. Using the Bayesian approach with these prior distributions will provide numerically nearly identical point and interval estimates as the frequentist approach. However, the Bayesian approach also allows for a wide variety of other prior distributions. Since exact values for the constrained parameters are seldom if ever known,

the consideration of nondegenerate prior distributions covering a range of values is more realistic.

This idea, to use a prior distribution to honestly represent uncertainty, rather than fixing the quantity at hand in order to gain identification, has been repeatedly and forcefully argued for by Sander Greenland. For instance, Greenland (2003, p. 53) includes:

Model expansion to include unidentified bias parameters is an attempt to introduce some realism into conventional sampling models.

While Greenland (2009a, p. 1662) says:

The approach illustrates how conventional analyses depend on implicit certainty that bias parameters are null and how these implausible assumptions can be replaced by plausible priors for bias parameters.

Then later in the same work (pp. 1670–1671):

In summary, a major problem with conventional frequentist and Bayesian analyses is that they conceal dogmatic point-null priors on hidden bias parameters. Bias analysis is not limited to such overoptimistic extremes. It thus frees researchers from having to use the ludicrous priors implicit in conventional results, and shows how classic validity problems can be subsumed under the topic of analysis with missing data. I thus advocate that bias modelling be covered in basic statistical training in the health sciences, and that epidemiologists understand principles of bias analysis so that they fully appreciate the complexity of inference from observational data.

Similar sentiments are found in Greenland (2009b, p. 195):

In designed experiments and surveys, known laws or design features provide checks on the most relevant aspects of a model and identify the target parameters. In contrast, in most observational studies in the health and social sciences, the primary study data do not identify and may not even bound target parameters. Discrepancies between target and analogous identified parameters (biases) are then of paramount concern, which forces a major shift in modeling strategies. Conventional approaches are based on conditional testing of equality constraints, which correspond to implausible point-mass priors. When these constraints are not identified by available data, however, no such testing is possible. In response, implausible constraints can be relaxed into penalty functions derived from plausible prior distributions.

Greenland also has much to offer on the issue that "owning up" to a lack of identification has profound implications for how evidence accumulates with sample size. For instance, in (Greenland, 2005, p. 287) he wrote:

'Collect better data' becomes a relevant slogan when it is feasible to do so. Multiple-bias modelling is then a useful ally in making clear that the added value of more observations of previous quality (e.g., case-control studies with unknown and possibly large amounts of bias) is much less than conventional statistical formulae convey ... Conventional standard errors shrink to 0 as the number of observations increases, and total uncertainty approaches the combined bias uncertainty. At some point, mere replication or enlargement of observational studies is not cost effective, and innovations to reduce bias are essential.

The quite recent literature contains a diversity of opinions about Bayesian inference in partially identified settings. For instance, San Martın and González (2010, p. 77) express concern that the posterior mean of the target parameter is identically the posterior mean of a different target expressed in terms of the embedded identified model. That is, in our notation, the posterior mean of $g(\phi, \lambda)$ is identically the posterior mean of $g_\pi(\phi)$. On this matter they say:

From a practical point of view, this means that if an unidentified parameter is estimated by its posterior distribution, the users should be warned that this estimate does not provide any updating of the unidentified parameter, but only of the identified parameter. This is more relevant when the unidentified parameter is a parameter of interest. In this case, if such a warning is not explicit, erroneous conclusions can be drawn from the analysis, namely, it can be concluded that information about the unidentified parameter has been obtained, when in reality the only information that is obtained is about the identified parameter.

In their investigations, Moon and Schorfheide (2012, p. 780) are also somewhat negative, citing concern about sensitivity to the choice of prior distribution. With slight adaptation to match present notation, they say.

The Bayesian approach induces a probability distribution across the identified set conditional on ϕ. This distribution is not updated through the likelihood function and creates a challenge for the reporting of Bayesian inference. In this regard, it is important to report estimates of the identified set as well as the conditional prior for $(\psi^* | \phi^* = \hat{\phi})$ along with Bayesian posteriors so that the audience can assess whether, due to the choice of prior, the posterior concentrates in a small subset of the identified set.

However, in line with some of the thoughts in Gustafson (2014) about the shape of the LPD over the identification region, Liao and Jiang (2010, p. 278) express a more positive sentiment:

However, we point out that a posterior density provides more information than a region estimation since it can also incorporate prior information and describe how likely the true parameter is to be distributed both inside and outside the identified region.

Finally, the autobiographical remarks of Manski (2010, p. 14) make for extremely interesting reading. In the context of the econometrics community, he reports experiencing considerable historical resistance to his work on partial identification:

> Econometricians and empirical workers long considered partial identification to be a curious "niche" topic distant from the mainstream. Some viewed the topic with considerable hostility. Why so? ... One problem was that many researchers were (and continue to be) much more comfortable with building on existing literature than with unlearning and discovery. As a general matter, researchers often find it psychologically difficult or even impossible to question received wisdom and go back to basics. In the present case, the received wisdom was that identification is an all-or-nothing proposition, with available data and maintained assumptions either fully revealing a population parameter or revealing nothing at all. There is no logical reason to think this, and scattered examples of partial identification were shown as long ago as the 1930s. Nevertheless, econometricians and empirical researchers were long fixated on what we now call point identification.

This sentiment likely rings true amongst the relatively small number of researchers who have grappled with partial identification in their work. It certainly does with this author!

8.2   What is the Road ahead?

Having looked back at thoughts and perceptions concerning Bayesian inference in partially identified models, we now turn to the future. It seems that work remains to be done across the whole spectrum of theory, methods, and applications.

On the theory and methods side, as evidenced in this book, we can get a good handle on partial identification in problems where we can identify a transparent parameterization. There is a serious bottleneck, however, in getting beyond this class of problems. In part this is a theory bottleneck, since given a complicated model we have no completely general strategies for determining whether or not it is fully identified. And, even if we are convinced it is only partially identified, without a transparent parameterization we have no general strategies to understand the extent to which data can inform target parameters. A point stressed in Section 7.1 is that this is also a methods bottleneck. Say we had widely robust black-box algorithms to compute posterior distributions, without a tendency to be problematic when faced with nonidentified models. Then we could simply observe posterior distributions arising from simulated datasets of various sizes. However, we do not have such algorithms. Thus theory and methods research breakthroughs are sorely needed in order to confidently hone our understanding of more complex partially identified models.

On the applied side, a good portion of what is needed seems to be "preaching." There remains a tendency (or a "fixation" as Manski (2010) put it) amongst statisticians to think of identification in very polarized terms. That is, an identified model is good and can be used, a nonidentified model is bad and should not be used. And, again appealing to Manski's thoughts, we are not rushing to "unlearn" this dogma. As best he can recall, the present author went through his graduate statistical education without ever seeing an example of inference in a partially identified setting, and he suspects this is still true for most students today.

In closing then, it seems appropriate to summarize the sermon:

• Identification is nuanced. Its absence does not preclude a parameter being well estimated, nor does its presence guarantee a parameter can be well estimated.

• If we really took limitations of study designs and data quality seriously, then partially identified problems would crop up all the time in a variety of scientific fields.

• Making modeling assumptions for the sole purpose of gaining full identification can be a mug's game. If the assumption in question is not defensible for a given application, then one may simply be replacing estimator bias due to lack of identification with bias due to model misspecification. And, worse than that, interval estimates that acknowledge bias due to lack of identification will be replaced by interval estimates not acknowledging model misspecification, i.e., intervals that imbue false confidence.

• If we accept partial identification, then consequently we need to regard sample size differently. There are profound implications of posterior variance tending to a positive limit as the sample size grows.

Here endeth the lesson. Please join me in spreading the word!

Bibliography

Aldrich, J. (2002), 'How likelihood and identification went Bayesian', *International Statistical Review* **70**, 79–98.

Barankin, E. W. (1960), 'Sufficient parameters: Solution of the minimal dimensionality problem', *Annals of the Institute of Mathematical Statistics* **12**, 91–118.

Berger, J. O. (1985), *Statistical Decision Theory and Bayesian Analysis*, Springer.

Bernardo, J. M. and Smith, A. F. M. (1994), *Bayesian Theory*, Wiley.

Bolstad, W. M. (2007), *Introduction to Bayesian Statistics*, 2nd edn, Wiley.

Burstyn, I., Kim, H.-M., Yasui, Y. and Cherry, N. M. (2009), 'The virtues of a deliberately misspecified disease model in demonstrating a gene-environment interaction', *Occupational and Environmental Medicine* **66**, 374–380.

Carlin, B. P. and Louis, T. A. (2011), *Bayesian Methods for Data Analysis*, 3rd edn, Chapman & Hall, CRC Press.

Carroll, R. J., Ruppert, D., Stefanski, L. A. and Crainiceanu, C. M. (2006), *Measurement Error in Nonlinear Models: A Modern Perspective*, 2nd edn, Chapman & Hall, CRC Press.

Chatterjee, N. and Carroll, R. (2005), 'Semiparametric maximum likelihood estimation exploiting gene-environment independence in case-control studies', *Biometrika* **92**, 399–418.

Chen, H. and Chen, J. (2011), 'On information coded in gene-environment independence in case-control studies', *American Journal of Epidemiology* **174**, 736–743.

Chickering, D. and Pearl, J. (1996), A clinician's tool for analyzing non-compliance, *in* 'Proceedings of the Thirteenth National Conference on Artificial Intelligence (AAAI-96), Portland, OR', Vol. 2, pp. 1269–1276.

Christensen, R., Johnson, W. O., Branscum, A. J. and Hanson, T. E. (2011), *Bayesian Ideas and Data Analysis: An Introduction for Scientists and Statisticians*, Chapman & Hall, CRC Press.

Cook, S., Gelman, A. and Rubin, D. B. (2006), 'Validation of software for

Bayesian models using posterior quantiles', *Journal of Computational and Graphical Statistics* **15**, 675–692.

Dawid, A. (1979), 'Conditional independence in statistical theory', *Journal of the Royal Statistical Society, Series B* **41**, 1–31.

Dendukuri, N., Bélisle, P. and Joseph, L. (2010), 'Bayesian sample size for diagnostic test studies in the absence of a gold standard: Comparing identifiable with non-identifiable models', *Statistics in Medicine* **29**, 2688–2697.

Dendukuri, N., Rahme, E., Bélisle, P. and Joseph, L. (2004), 'Bayesian sample size determination for prevalence and diagnostic test studies in the absence of a gold standard test', *Biometrics* **60**, 388–397.

Doucet, A., De Freitas, N., Gordon, N. et al. (2001), *Sequential Monte Carlo Methods in Practice*, Vol. 1, Springer.

Frangakis, C. E. and Rubin, D. B. (2002), 'Principal stratification in causal inference', *Biometrics* **58**, 21–29.

Fréchet, M. (1951), 'Sur les tableaux de corrélation dont les marges sont données', *Annales de l'Université de Lyon, Section A* **9**, 53–77.

Gelfand, A. and Smith, A. (1990), 'Sampling-based approaches to calculating marginal densities', *Journal of the American Statistical Association* **85**, 398–409.

Gelman, A., Carlin, J. B., Stern, H. S., Dunson, D. B., Vehtari, A. and Rubin, D. B. (2013), *Bayesian Data Analysis*, Chapman & Hall, CRC Press.

Ghosal, S. (1996), A review of consistency and convergence rates of posterior distributions, *in* 'Proceedings of Varanashi Symposium in Bayesian Inference', Banaras Hindu University.

Gile, K. J. and Handcock, M. S. (2010), 'Respondent-driven sampling: An assessment of current methodology', *Sociological Methodology* **40**, 285–327.

Goetghebeur, E., Liinev, J., Boelaert, M. and Van der Stuyft, P. (2000), 'Diagnostic test analyses in search of their gold standard: Latent class analyses with random effects', *Statistical Methods in Medical Research* **9**, 231–248.

Goodman, L. A. (1974), 'Exploratory latent structure analysis using both identifiable and unidentifiable models', *Biometrika* **61**, 215–231.

Greenland, S. (2000), 'An introduction to instrumental variables for epidemiologists', *International Journal of Epidemiology* **29**, 722–729.

Greenland, S. (2003), 'The impact of prior distributions for uncontrolled confounding and response bias: A case study of the relation of wire codes and magnetic fields to childhood leukemia', *Journal of the American Statistical Association* **98**, 47–55.

Greenland, S. (2005), 'Multiple-bias modelling for analysis of observational data', *Journal of the Royal Statistical Society, Series A* **168**, 267–306.

Greenland, S. (2009a), 'Bayesian perspectives for epidemiological research: III. Bias analysis via missing data methods', *International Journal of Epidemiology* **38**, 1662–1673.

Greenland, S. (2009b), 'Relaxation penalties and priors for plausible modeling of nonidentified bias sources', *Statistical Science* **24**, 195–210.

Gustafson, P. (2005a), 'On model expansion, model contraction, identifiability, and prior information: two illustrative scenarios involving mismeasured variables (with discussion)', *Statistical Science* **20**, 111–140.

Gustafson, P. (2005b), 'The utility of prior information and stratification for parameter estimation with two screening tests but no gold standard', *Statistics in Medicine* **24**, 1203–1217.

Gustafson, P. (2006), 'Sample size implications when biases are modelled rather than ignored', *Journal of the Royal Statistical Society, Series A* **169**, 883–902.

Gustafson, P. (2007), 'Measurement error modeling with an approximate instrumental variable', *Journal of the Royal Statistical Society, Series B* **69**, 797–815.

Gustafson, P. (2009), 'What are the limits of posterior distributions arising from nonidentified models, and why should we care?', *Journal of the American Statistical Association* **104**, 1682–1695.

Gustafson, P. (2010), 'Bayesian inference for partially identified models', *International Journal of Biostatistics* **6**, issue 2 article 17.

Gustafson, P. (2011), Comment on 'Transparent parameterizations of models for potential outcomes,' by Richardson, Evans, and Robins, *in* J. M. Bernardo, M. J. Bayarri, J. O. Berger, A. P. Dawid, D. Heckerman, A. F. M. Smith and M. West, eds, 'Bayesian Statistics 9: Proceedings of the Ninth Valencia International Meeting', Oxford University Press.

Gustafson, P. (2012), 'On the behaviour of bayesian credible intervals in partially identified models', *Electronic Journal of Statistics* **6**, 2107–2124.

Gustafson, P. (2014), 'Bayesian inference in partially identified models: Is the shape of the posterior distribution useful?', *Electronic Journal of Statistics* **8**, 476–496.

Gustafson, P. and Burstyn, I. (2011), '"Bayesian inference of gene-environment interaction from incomplete data: What happens when information on environment is disjoint from data on gene and disease?', *Statistics in Medicine* **30**, 877–889.

Gustafson, P., Gilbert, M., Xia, M., Michelow, W., Robert, W., Trussler, T., McGuire, M., Paquette, D., Moore, D. M. and Gustafson, R. (2013), 'Impact of statistical adjustment for frequency of venue attendance in a venue-based survey of men who have sex with men', *American Journal of Epidemiology* **177**, 1157–1164.

Gustafson, P. and Greenland, S. (2006), 'The performance of random co-efficient regression in accounting for residual confounding', *Biometrics* **62**, 760–768.

Gustafson, P. and Greenland, S. (2009), 'Interval estimation for messy observational data', *Statistical Science* **24**, 328–342.

Gustafson, P., Le, N. D. and Saskin, R. (2001), 'Case-control analysis with partial knowledge of exposure misclassification probabilities', *Biometrics* **57**, 598–609.

Gustafson, P., McCandless, L. C., Levy, A. R. and Richardson, S. (2010), 'Simplified Bayesian sensitivity analysis for mismeasured and unobserved confounders', *Biometrics* **66**, 1129–1137.

Hanson, T. and Johnson, W. (2005), 'Comment on 'On model expansion, model contraction, identifiability and prior information: Two illustrative scenarios involving mismeasured variables,' by Gustafson', *Statistical Science* **20**, 131–134.

Hastings, W. K. (1970), 'Monte Carlo sampling methods using Markov chains and their applications', *Biometrika* **57**, 97–109.

Hernán, M. A. and Robins, J. M. (2006), 'Instruments for causal inference: an epidemiologist's dream?', *Epidemiology* **17**, 360–372.

Hoff, P. D. (2009), *A First Course in Bayesian Statistical Methods*, Springer.

Hopper, J. L. and Seeman, E. (1994), 'The bone density of female twins discordant for tobacco use', *New England Journal of Medicine* **330**, 387–392.

Huber, P. (1967), The behavior of maximum likelihood estimates under non-standard conditions, *in* 'Proceedings of the fifth Berkeley symposium on mathematical statistics and probability', Vol. 1, pp. 221–233.

Hui, S. L. and Walter, S. D. (1980), 'Estimating the error rates of diagnostic tests', *Biometrics* **36**, 167–171.

Hui, S. L. and Zhou, X. H. (1998), 'Evaluation of diagnostic tests without gold standards', *Statistical Methods in Medical Research* **7**, 354–370.

Imbens, G. W. and Manski, C. F. (2004), 'Confidence intervals for partially identified parameters', *Econometrica* **72**, 1845–1857.

Imbens, G. W. and Rubin, D. B. (1997), 'Bayesian inference for causal effects in randomized experiments with noncompliance', *Annals of Statistics* **25**, 305–327.

Johnston, L. G. and Sabin, K. (2010), 'Sampling hard-to-reach populations with respondent driven sampling', *Methodological Innovations Online* **5**, 38–48.

Jones, G., Johnson, W. O., Hanson, T. E. and Christensen, R. (2010), 'Identifiability of models for multiple diagnostic testing in the absence of a gold standard', *Biometrics* **66**, 855–863.

Joseph, L. and Bélisle, P. (2013), 'Bayesian sample size determination for case-control studies when exposure may be misclassified', *American Journal of Epidemiology* **178**, 1673–1679.

Joseph, L., Gyorkos, T. and Coupal, L. (1995), 'Bayesian estimation of disease prevalence and the parameters of diagnostic tests in the absence of a gold standard', *American Journal of Epidemiology* **141**, 263–272.

Kadane, J. B. (1974), The role of identification in Bayesian theory, *in* S. E. Fienberg and A. Zellner, eds, 'Studies in Bayesian Econometrics and Statistics, In Honor of Leonard J. Savage', p. 175.

Karon, J. M. and Wejnert, C. (2012), 'Statistical methods for the analysis of time–location sampling data', *Journal of Urban Health* **89**, 565–586.

King, G. (2013), *A solution to the ecological inference problem: Reconstructing individual behavior from aggregate data*, Princeton University Press.

Kosinski, A. S. and Flanders, W. D. (1999), 'Evaluating the exposure and disease relationship with adjustment for different types of exposure misclassification: a regression approach', *Statistics in Medicine* **18**, 2795–2808.

Kraft, P., Yen, Y.-C., Stram, D. O., Morrison, J. and Gauderman, W. J. (2007), 'Exploiting gene-environment interaction to detect genetic associations', *Human Heredity* **63**, 111–119.

Lash, T. L., Fox, M. P. and Fink, A. K. (2009), *Applying Quantitative Bias Analysis to Epidemiologic Data*, Springer.

Lawlor, D. A., Harbord, R. M., Sterne, J. A., Timpson, N. and Davey Smith, G. (2008), 'Mendelian randomization: using genes as instruments for making causal inferences in epidemiology', *Statistics in Medicine* **27**, 1133–1163.

Lee, P. M. (2012), *Bayesian Statistics: An Introduction*, 4th edn, Wiley.

Liao, Y. and Jiang, W. (2010), 'Bayesian analysis in moment inequality models', *Annals of Statistics* **38**, 275–316.

Lindley, D. V. (1972), *Bayesian Statistics: A Review*, Society for Industrial and Applied Mathematics.

Little, R. J. A. and Rubin, D. B. (2002), *Statistical Analysis with Missing Data*, 2nd edn, Wiley.

Lumley, T. (2004), 'Analysis of complex survey samples', *Journal of Statistical Software* **9**, 1–19.

Lunn, D., Spiegelhalter, D., Thomas, A. and Best, N. (2009), 'The BUGS project: Evolution, critique and future directions', *Statistics in Medicine* **28**, 3049–3067.

Lunn, D., Thomas, A., Best, N. and Spiegelhalter, D. (2000), 'WinBUGS-a Bayesian modelling framework: Concepts, structure, and extensibility', *Statistics and Computing* **10**, 325–337.

Luo, H., Burstyn, I. and Gustafson, P. (2013), 'Investigations of gene-disease associations: Costs and benefits of environmental data', *Epidemiology* **24**, 562–568.

Manski, C. F. (2003), *Partial Identification of Probability Distributions*, Springer.

Manski, C. F. (2010), 'Unlearning and discovery', *American Economist* **55**, 9–18.

McCandless, L. C., Gustafson, P. and Levy, A. R. (2007), 'Bayesian sensitivity analysis for unmeasured confounding in observational studies', *Statistics in Medicine* **26**, 2331–2347.

McCandless, L. C., Gustafson, P. and Levy, A. R. (2008), 'A sensitivity analysis using information about measured confounders yielded improved assessments of uncertainty from unmeasured confounding', *Journal of Clinical Epidemiology* **61**, 247–255.

McCandless, L. C., Gustafson, P., Levy, A. R. and Richardson, S. (2012), 'Hierarchical priors for bias parameters in Bayesian sensitivity analysis for unmeasured confounding', *Statistics in Medicine* **31**, 383–396.

M'Lan, C. E., Joseph, L. and Wolfson, D. B. (2006), 'Bayesian sample size determination for case-control studies', *Journal of the American Statistical Association* **101**, 760–772.

Moon, H. R. and Schorfheide, F. (2012), 'Bayesian and frequentist inference in partially identified models', *Econometrica* **80**, 755–782.

Morgenstern, H. (1995), 'Ecologic studies in epidemiology: Concepts, principles, and methods', *Annual Review of Public Health* **16**, 61–81.

Neath, A. and Samaniego, F. (1997), 'On the efficacy of Bayesian inference for nonidentifiable models', *American Statistician* **51**, 225–232.

Newhouse, J. P. and McClellan, M. (1998), 'Econometrics in outcomes research: the use of instrumental variables', *Annual Review of Public Health* **19**, 17–34.

Palatini, P., Pessina, A. and Dal Palù, C. (1993), 'The hypertension and ambulatory recording venetia study (harvest): a trial on the predictive value of ambulatory blood pressure monitoring for the development of fixed hypertension in patients with borderline hypertension', *High Blood Pressure* **2**, 11–18.

Pasek, J., with some assistance from Alex Tahk and some code modified from R-core (2012), *weights: Weighting and Weighted Statistics*. R package version 0.75.
URL: *http://CRAN.R-project.org/package=weights*

Pearl, J. (2000), *Causality: Models, Reasoning, and Inference*, Cambridge University Press.

Pepe, M. S. and Janes, H. (2007), 'Insights into latent class analysis of diagnostic test performance', *Biostatistics* **8**, 474–484.

Poirier, D. (1998), 'Revising beliefs in nonidentified models', *Econometric Theory* **14**, 483–509.

Qu, Y., Tan, M. and Kutner, M. H. (1996), 'Random effects models in latent class analysis for evaluating accuracy of diagnostic tests', *Biometrics* **52**, 797–810.

Rahme, E., Joseph, L. and Gyorkos, T. W. (2000), 'Bayesian sample size determination for estimating binomial parameters from data subject to misclassification', *Journal of the Royal Statistical Society: Series C* **49**, 119–128.

Rassen, J. A., Brookhart, M. A., Glynn, R. J., Mittleman, M. A. and Schneeweiss, S. (2009), 'Instrumental variables I: Instrumental variables exploit natural variation in nonexperimental data to estimate causal relationships', *Journal of Clinical Epidemiology* **62**, 1226–1232.

Richardson, T. S., Evans, R. J. and Robins, J. M. (2011), Transparent parameterizations of models for potential outcomes, *in* J. M. Bernardo, M. J. Bayarri, J. O. Berger, A. P. Dawid, D. Heckerman, A. F. M. Smith and M. West, eds, 'Bayesian Statistics 9: Proceedings of the Ninth Valencia International Meeting', Oxford University Press, pp. 569–610.

Romano, J. P. and Shaikh, A. M. (2008), 'Inference for identifiable parameters in partially identified econometric models', *Journal of Statistical Planning and Inference* **138**, 2786–2807.

Rosin, M. P., Cheng, X., Poh, C., Lam, W. L., Huang, Y., Lovas, J., Berean, K., Epstein, J. B., Priddy, R., Le, N. D. et al. (2000), 'Use of allelic loss to predict malignant risk for low-grade oral epithelial dysplasia', *Clinical Cancer Research* **6**, 357–362.

Rosner, B. (2000), *Fundamentals of Biostatistics*, 5th edn, Duxbury Press.

Rothenberg, T. J. (1971), 'Identification in parametric models', *Econometrica* **39**, 577–591.

Sacerdote, C., Guarrera, S., Smith, G. D., Grioni, S., Krogh, V., Masala, G., Mattiello, A., Palli, D., Panico, S., Tumino, R. et al. (2007), 'Lactase persistence and bitter taste response: instrumental variables and Mendelian randomization in epidemiologic studies of dietary factors and cancer risk', *American Journal of Epidemiology* **166**, 576–581.

San Martın, E. and González, J. (2010), 'Bayesian identifiability: Contributions to an inconclusive debate', *Chilean Journal of Statistics* **1**, 69–91.

Schork, M. A. and Remington, R. D. (2000), *Statistics with Applications to the Biological and Health Sciences*, Prentice Hall.

Semaan, S. (2010), 'Time-space sampling and respondent-driven sampling with hard-to-reach populations', *Methodological Innovations Online* **5**, 60–75.

Shapiro, A. (1986), 'Asymptotic theory of overparameterized structural models', *Journal of the American Statistical Association* **81**, 142–149.

Smith, G. D. and Ebrahim, S. (2003), 'Mendelian randomization: Can genetic epidemiology contribute to understanding environmental determinants of disease?', *International Journal of Epidemiology* **32**, 1–22.

Smith, G. D. and Ebrahim, S. (2004), 'Mendelian randomization: prospects, potentials, and limitations', *International Journal of Epidemiology* **33**, 30–42.

Stamey, J. D., Seaman, J. W. and Young, D. M. (2005), 'Bayesian sample-size determination for inference on two binomial populations with no gold standard classifier', *Statistics in Medicine* **24**, 2963–2976.

Stan Development Team (2013), 'Stan: A c++ library for probability and sampling, version 1.3'.
URL: *http://mc-stan.org/*

Steenland, K. and Greenland, S. (2004), 'Monte-Carlo sensitivity analysis and Bayesian analysis of smoking as an unmeasured confounder in a study of silica and lung cancer', *American Journal of Epidemiology* **160**, 384–392.

Stoye, J. (2009), 'More on confidence intervals for partially identified parameters', *Econometrica* **77**, 1299–1315.

Sturges, H. A. (1926), 'The choice of a class interval', *Journal of the American Statistical Association* **21**, 65–66.

Szpiro, A. A., Rice, K. M. and Lumley, T. (2010), 'Model-robust regression and a Bayesian sandwich estimator', *Annals of Applied Statistics* **4**, 2099–2113.

Tierney, L. (1994), 'Markov chains for exploring posterior distributions', *Annals of Statistics* **22**, 1701–1728.

Umbach, D. and Weinberg, C. (1998), 'Designing and analysing case-control studies to exploit independence of genotype and exposure', *Statistics in Medicine* **16**, 1731–1743.

Vansteelandt, S., Goetghebeur, E., Kenward, M. G. and Molenberghs, G. (2006), 'Ignorance and uncertainty regions as inferential tools in a sensitivity analysis', *Statistica Sinica* **16**, 953–979.

Wakefield, J. (2004), 'Ecological inference for 2× 2 tables (with discussion)', *Journal of the Royal Statistical Society, Series A* **167**, 385–445.

Wakefield, J. (2008), 'Ecologic studies revisited', *Annual Review of Public Health* **29**, 75–90.

Wang, D., Shen, T. and Gustafson, P. (2012), 'Partial identification arising from nondifferential exposure misclassification: How informative are data on the unlikely, maybe, and likely exposed?', *International Journal of Biostatistics* **8**, issue 1, article 31.

Wang, F. and Gelfand, A. E. (2002), 'A simulation-based approach to Bayesian sample size determination for performance under a given model and for separating models', *Statistical Science* **17**, 193–208.

White, H. (1982), 'Maximum likelihood estimation of misspecified models', *Econometrica* **50**, 1–25.

Xia, M. and Gustafson, P. (2012), 'A Bayesian method for estimating prevalence in the presence of a hidden sub-population', *Statistics in Medicine* **31**, 2386–2398.

Xia, M. and Gustafson, P. (2014), 'Bayesian sensitivity analyses for hidden sub-populations in weighted sampling', *Canadian Journal of Statistics* **42**, 436–450.

Index